APPLETON & LANGE'S REVIEW FOR THE
SURGICAL TECHNOLOGY
EXAMINATION

SECOND EDITION

DEANNA CLOUSE
MAY 1988

APPLETON & LANGE'S REVIEW FOR THE

SURGICAL TECHNOLOGY EXAMINATION

SECOND EDITION

Edited by

Nancy M. Allmers, R.N., B.A., M.A.
Director, Surgical Technology Program
Bergen Community College
Paramus, New Jersey

Joan Ann Verderame, R.N., B.A., M.A.
Instructor, Surgical Technology Program
Bergen Community College
Paramus, New Jersey

**Appleton
&Lange**
Norwalk, Connecticut/Los Altos, California

Dedicated
to our students
past, present, and future

0-8385-0215-6

Notice: The author(s) and publisher of this volume have taken care that the information and recommendations contained herein are accurate and compatible with the standards generally accepted at the time of publication.

87 88 89 90 91 / 10 9 8 7 6 5 4 3 2 1

Prentice-Hall of Australia, Pty. Ltd., Sydney
Prentice-Hall Canada, Inc.
Prentice-Hall Hispanoamericana, S.A., Mexico
Prentice-Hall of India Private Limited, New Delhi
Prentice-Hall International (UK) Limited, London
Prentice-Hall of Japan, Inc., Tokyo
Prentice-Hall of Southeast Asia (Pte.) Ltd., Singapore
Whitehall Books Ltd., Wellington, New Zealand
Editora Prentice-Hall do Brasil Ltda., Rio de Janeiro

Library of Congress Cataloging-in-Publication Data

Allmers, Nancy M.
  Appleton & Lange's review for the surgical technology examination.

  Rev. ed. of: Surgical technology examination review.
  Bibliography: p.
  1. Surgical technology – Examinations, questions, etc.
I. Verderame, Joan Ann. II. Allmers, Nancy M.
Surgical technology examination review. III. Title.
IV. Title: Appleton and Lange's review for the surgical
technology examination. V. Title: Review for the surgical
technology examination. [DNLM: 1. Operating Room
Technicians – examination questions. WY 18 A439s]
RD32.3.A45   1987   617'.91'0076   86-32239
ISBN 0-8385-0215-6

PRINTED IN THE UNITED STATES OF AMERICA

Contents

Preface

Review for the Surgical Technology Examination, second edition, has been designed to assist technicians planning to take the National Certification Exam for Surgical Technologists, which is given every March and September. Although unable to guarantee a perfect score, a study guide can provide a good deal of assistance in test preparation by enabling the student to review relevant material while becoming familiar with the type of questions that will be encountered on the exam.

The ever-growing body of knowledge necessary to prepare the surgical technologist for a professional role in the operating room requires that competency be measured by an exam that tests both constant and technologically up-to-date information.

With this in mind, the authors have prepared a second edition of the review book that has been extensively revised and updated to include those advances in technology that have emerged in the last 4 years.

The book contains over 1500 questions that closely correlate in percentage the amount prescribed in the Study Guide for Certification provided by the Liaison Council of the Association of Surgical Technologists. The text is divided into five areas of concentration. Each section is further divided into subsections, Surgical Procedures – Orthopedics. Each question has one answer, a full-length explanation and a reference note for further study in the area. Difficulty in a single area indicates a need for individual study emphasis.

Upon completion of the review, you are encouraged to take the Practice Test, which closely parallels the national exam. The exam questions are randomly selected to provide the student with a composite of questions that may appear on an actual exam. Although the questions are not from an actual certifying exam, they typify the type and style of question that may appear on the test.

Acknowledgments

We express our gratitude to a postgraduate of our program, Laura Wallin, C.S.T., for her excellent drawings.

Introduction

ORGANIZATION OF THE BOOK

The book is organized into five major sections, which are the major topic areas covered on the Certifying Examination for Surgical Technologists:

1. Basic Sciences (including Terminology, Anatomy and Physiology, Microbiology, Pharmacology, Wound Healing and Gross Anatomy)
2. Patient Care (including Pre-Op Routine, Transportation, Positioning, Related Nursing Procedures, and Medical/Legal Aspects)
3. Aseptic Technique and Environmental Control (including Sterilization, Disinfection, and Antisepsis; Packaging and Dispensing of Supplies; Environmental Control; and Aseptic Technique in General Procedures)
4. Supplies and Equipment (including Classification of Sutures and Needles; Classification of Instruments; Dressing and Packings; Catheters, Drains, Tubes, and Collecting Mechanisms; and Equipment)
5. Surgical Procedures (including General Surgery; Gynecologic Procedures; EENT and Plastic Surgery; Genitourinary Procedures; Thoracic, Cardiovascular, and Peripheral Vascular Procedures; Orthopedics and Plaster; and Neurosurgery)

Each section is designed to facilitate your review of the major content areas of surgical technology. In each section you are given ample practice at honing your question-taking skills. In addition, because each group of questions is preceded by a heading that identifies the particular subspecialty area (e.g., Basic Sciences – Terminology), you are able to test your current knowledge in each of these areas.

Finally, each section ends with detailed explanations of each question for reinforcement of knowledge. Each of these explanations is referenced to a specific page in a text or journal so that you can supplement your studying with further reading.

After all the individual review sections, there is an integrated Practice Test, which will enable you to assess your areas of strength and weakness under simulated exam conditions.

HOW TO ANSWER A QUESTION INTELLIGENTLY

Unlike many examinations, which are a composite of several multiple-choice question types, the National Certification Exam for Surgical Technologists uses only one major type of question. Each question will have a "stem," which presents a problem or asks a question. The stem is then followed by *four* choices, only one of which is entirely correct. "Distractors," which are the choices other than the correct answer, may be partially correct; however, there can only be one *best* answer.

Although the question type is constant within the exam, the degree of difficulty may vary. Some questions require rote memory, some require problem solving, and others require evaluation and judgment. When the stem of the question takes on a negative aspect, the word "no" or "except" will be printed in italics to catch your eye and remind you that the correct answer will be the exception to the statement in the stem of the question.

Sample Question 1

A left subcostal incision indicates surgery of the

    A. gallbladder
    B. pancreas
    C. spleen
    D. common bile duct

This question could be answered from rote memory, placing the term "subcostal" with the anatomic structure "spleen." It is more likely that the student will conjure up a picture of the human abdomen and discount gallbladder (choice A) and common bile duct (choice D) immediately because they are located on the right side of the abdominal cavity. Thus, two choices are ruled out as possible answers, improving the odds of selecting the correct answer from 25 to 50%. Although the tail of the pancreas reaches over to the left side of the body and is adjacent to the spleen, spleen is clearly the best choice and the only correct answer.

TABLE 1. STRATEGIES FOR ANSWERING QUESTIONS*

1. Remember that only one choice can be the correct answer.
2. Read the question carefully to be sure that you understand what is being asked.
3. Quickly read each choice for familiarity. (This important step is often not done by test takers.)
4. Go back and consider each choice individually.
5. If a choice is partially correct, tentatively consider it to be incorrect. (This step will help you lessen your choices and increase your odds of choosing the correct choice/answer.)
6. Consider the remaining choices and select the one you think is the answer. At this point, you may want to quickly scan the stem to be sure you understand the question and your answer.
7. Fill in the appropriate circle on the answer sheet. (Even if you do not know the answer, you should at least guess—you are scored on the number of correct answers, so **do not leave any blanks.**)

*Note that steps 2 through 7 should take an average of 40 to 45 seconds total. The actual examination is timed for an average of 40 to 45 seconds per question.

Sample Question 2

An elderly female, sleeping soundly, arrives in the OR via stretcher with siderails in place and safety strap intact. She is placed alone outside of her assigned OR. The woman wakens, climbs off the stretcher and receives a deep scalp laceration. The circulating nurse

    A. can be charged with abandonment
    B. can be charged with simple assault
    C. can be charged with battery
    D. cannot be charged because safety devices were in place

This question is more difficult. Although we clearly see (choices B & C) as incorrect because the nurse had no physical part in the injury to the patient, the difficulty is now in choosing between the remaining answers. Choice D may appear correct because the stem of the question tells us that *all* safety devices were intact. It is only with knowledge of the legal aspect of OR procedures that we know that the key word *alone* signifies culpability on the part of the nurse. Standard OR procedures claim that one is guilty of abandonment if a patient is left alone at any time when in the care of OR personnel, and may be charged as such in a court of law.

HOW TO USE THE BOOK

It will probably be the most efficient use of your time to follow the book from front to back, chapter to chapter, answering questions and noting difficult areas after completion of a section or subsection. Continual notation in this book or on a small notepad, which you should keep with your review book, of general areas as well as subspecialty areas will provide you with a quick review at the end of the chapter. This will help you determine those areas that require the most emphasis

for study and those areas that require only cursory review. Specific page references are provided at the end of each explanation. The numbers presented in parentheses refer to a particular text and page: e.g., (37:107) indicates that the information can be found on page 107 of reference number 37 in the Bibliography. Jot down the references most commonly cited in that chapter. Most of the references are texts that are readily available at your nearest library.

When you have completed the review and any additional study that is necessary, you will be ready for the 250-question Practice Test located on page 147. The Practice Test is a unique feature of this book as it provides you with an assessment of your readiness in all sections covered by the actual National Certifying Exam.

As you may already know, the Certifying Exam integrates subtopics; i.e., the questions are not separated into discrete categories. Thus, you can use the Practice Test to acclimate yourself to taking this heterogeneous mixture of question topics. In addition, the Practice Test will give you practice answering a large number of questions over an extended period of time (3 hours).

When you've completed the entire Practice Test, you can check off your incorrect answers in the answer section. A 75% (188 question correct) should be considered the minimum acceptable score on this test. In addition, you should check your answers against those given on the Practice Test Subject List on page 178. If you get less than 75% correct in any of the subject areas, you may want to supplement your studying with the references provided.

The official source of all information with respect to the exam is The Association of Surgical Technologists, Inc., Caller No. E, Littleton, Colorado 80120. Applications for and information about the exam can be obtained from the Examination Department at this address. **Remember:** for all official information on the exam, you should contact the A.S.T. at the address above.

CHAPTER 1

Basic Sciences
Questions

Directions: Each of the questions or incomplete statements below is followed by four suggested answers or completions. Select the best answer in each case.

A. TERMINOLOGY

1. The root word *glosso* means

A. mouth
B. tongue
C. gums
D. cheek

2. Choledochitis means

A. inflammation of the gallbladder
B. inflammation of the common bile duct
C. presence of a stone in the gallbladder
D. presence of a stone in the common bile duct

3. A term which means having a rapid onset, severe symptoms, and a short course is:

A. infectious
B. inflammatory
C. chronic
D. acute

4. The suffix *cyte* represents

A. the bladder
B. a cyst
C. a cell
D. a tumor

5. The submental region is located

A. at the base of the skull
B. above the eyebrows
C. about the ears
D. below the chin

6. The root word *meso* means

A. many
B. middle
C. large
D. small

7. The root word *pseudo* means

A. left
B. true
C. false
D. complete

8. The root word *aden* means

A. lymph
B. gland
C. joint
D. bone

9. PRN means

A. immediately
B. as directed
C. after meals
D. as necessary

10. NPO means

A. at night
B. in manner directed
C. nothing by mouth
D. as needed

11. Distal is a term that indicates a point

A. closer to the body
B. away from the body
C. in the center of the body
D. toward the head

12. The term proximal refers to a point

A. closer to the body
B. toward the lower portion of the body
C. away from the body
D. toward the head

13. The suffix *ectomy* refers to

A. incision of an organ
B. drainage of an organ
C. removal of an organ
D. viewing of an organ

14. The symbol gtt means

A. drop
B. dose
C. mixture
D. solution

15. *Endo* means

A. within
B. outside
C. between
D. opposite

16. The appendix is located in the

A. RLQ
B. RUQ
C. LLQ
D. LUQ

17. Abduction means

A. movement away from median plane
B. movement toward median plane
C. movement superiorly
D. movement inferiorly

18. CO_2 represents

A. carbolic acid
B. carbohydrate
C. carbon dioxide
D. cobalt

19. The study of tumors is

A. otology
B. oncology
C. ophthalmology
D. radiology

20. The suffix added to a noun to denote pain is

A. *ic*
B. *algia*
C. *itis*
D. *ile*

21. The suffix *oma* denotes a/an

A. cyst
B. tumor
C. organ
D. lymph gland

22. The suffix *oscopy* means

A. opening into
B. drainage of
C. removal of
D. viewing of

23. A cc is equivalent to a

A. ml
B. cm
C. gtt
D. gr

24. Stricture is synonymous with

A. scar
B. stenosis
C. dilation
D. adhesion

25. The suffix *lysis* means

A. pathologic state
B. reduction of
C. motion
D. sensation

26. The root word *brady* means

A. fast
B. slow
C. short
D. long

27. Intravenous fluids are measured in

A. ml
B. cm
C. min
D. mm

28. The prefix *contra* means

A. around
B. against
C. with
D. away from

29. PID refers to inflammatory disease of

A. pelvic organs
B. vessels
C. brain
D. thoracic organs

30. A growth extending outward from a mucous membrane is a

A. diverticulum
B. cyst
C. polyp
D. ganglion

31. Dysuria is

A. scanty urination
B. painful urination
C. excessive urination
D. excess of urates in urines

32. The term denoting a hernia of the urinary bladder is

A. hydrocele
B. omphalocele
C. cystocele
D. varicocele

33. What term describes a disturbed kidney function that produces a toxic condition in the blood?

A. pyelonephritis
B. nephrosis
C. uremia
D. nephremia

34. Arteriosclerosis is

A. narrowing of an artery
B. necrosis of an artery
C. hardening of walls of arterioles
D. softening of arterial coats

35. Splenomegaly means

A. removal of the spleen
B. fixation of the spleen
C. an accessory spleen
D. enlargement of the spleen

36. The bodily function that denotes intestinal motility is called

A. digestion
B. enteroptosis
C. peristalsis
D. enteritis

37. The term profunda anatomically indicates

A. deep-seated
B. superior to
C. parallel to
D. in place of

38. Hypertrophy means

A. increase in size, in the context of cell size
B. decrease in size, in the context of cell size
C. increase in size, in the actual number of cells
D. decrease in size, in the actual number of cells

39. What is the antonym (opposite) of the prefix *ab*?

A. *an*
B. *ad*
C. *de*
D. *intra*

40. The root word *edem* indicates

A. dilation
B. swelling
C. feeling
D. pain

41. Which suffix is added to a term to express resemblance?

A. *osis*
B. *al*
C. *ous*
D. *oid*

42. An osteochondroma is a

A. bony tumor
B. tumor of bone and cartilage
C. fleshy tumor containing osseous tissue
D. tumor of fibrous and cartilaginous tissue

43. Flaccid means

A. lack of muscle tone
B. loss of function
C. wasted away
D. increase in muscle fiber size

44. Atrophy means

A. death of tissue
B. without contraction
C. wasting away
D. increase in muscle fiber size

45. The root word meaning tongue is

A. *lumbus*
B. *lingua*
C. *bucca*
D. *nucla*

46. All of the following are root words for blood *except*

A. *hema*
B. *hemato*
C. *homo*
D. *haemo*

47. A fossa is a

A. ridge
B. basinlike depression
C. projection
D. seam

48. Litho refers to a

A. tract
B. crack
C. stone
D. foreign body

49. An inch equals

A. 2.2 cm
B. 2.54 cm
C. 4.4 cm
D. 10 cm

50. The prefix *de* means

A. away from
B. to
C. of
D. through

51. Reduction in oxygen supply to the cells is

A. orthopnea
B. hypoxia
C. dyspnea
D. asphyxia

52. The directional term for near or on the back is

A. ventral
B. efferent
C. afferent
D. dorsal

53. When tissue is said to be necrotic, it is inferred that the tissue is

A. ischemic
B. inflamed
C. dead
D. contused

54. The prefix *supra* means

A. behind
B. under
C. above
D. before

55. The prefix *a* or *an* means

A. without
B. away from
C. toward
D. before

56. Painful menses is termed

A. dysuria
B. dysmenorrhea
C. amenorrhea
D. menorrhagia

57. The pigmented area surrounding the nipple is the

A. alveoli
B. areola
C. mammilla
D. sebaceous gland

58. Another term for gums is

A. crown
B. alveoli
C. gingiva
D. dentin

59. A clot that forms inside a vessel is known as a/an

A. infarct
B. aneurysm
C. embolus
D. thrombus

60. Bradycardia is

A. rapid pulse rate
B. rapid heart rate
C. irregular heart rate
D. slow pulse rate

61. Tachycardia is

A. rapid heart rate
B. irregular pulse rate
C. slow pulse rate
D. slow heart rate

62. Referred pain describes

A. pain that is sharp and cutting
B. pain that cannot be relieved easily
C. pain occurring along branches of a nerve
D. pain in an area other than its origin

63. Pain that cannot be easily relieved is called

A. intractable pain
B. acute pain
C. neuralgic pain
D. referred pain

64. A fluid-filled skin sac is a

A. wheal
B. papule
C. nodule
D. cyst

65. An open sore that does not heal is called a/an

A. urticaria
B. boil
C. ulcer
D. carbuncle

66. Which of the following is a nonmalignant tumor?

A. Ewing's tumor
B. fibroma
C. sarcoma
D. glioma

67. Muscular hypertrophy refers to

A. increase in the number of fibers
B. shortening of the muscle as it contracts
C. enlargement of muscle fibers
D. lengthening of the muscle as it contracts

68. What is a fissure in ano?

A. hemorrhoid
B. linear ulcer or crack on margin of anus
C. tubelike passageway near the anus
D. a groove in the temporal bone

69. Evulsion means

A. turning inside out
B. retroversion
C. tearing away of a part
D. incomplete

70. To what does dacryo refer?

A. eyelid
B. eyeball
C. cornea
D. lacrimal gland

B. ANATOMY AND PHYSIOLOGY

71. The hormone that regulates metabolism for the production of heat and energy in body tissue is

A. insulin
B. thyroxine   JODINE METABOLISM
C. progesterone
D. follicle-stimulating hormone

72. The adrenal glands are located

A. in the brain
B. above the kidney
C. in the pancreas
D. behind the thyroid gland

73. How many parathyroids are there in the body?

A. two
B. three
C. four
D. five

74. The islets of Langerhans are located in the

A. adrenals
B. parathyroids
C. pituitary
D. pancreas

75. All of the following are hormones produced in the anterior lobe of the pituitary gland *except*

A. somatotropic
B. gonadotropic
C. antidiuretic
D. lactogenic

76. Which gland is also known as the master gland?

A. thyroid
B. pituitary
C. adrenal
D. parathyroid

77. What substance must be in adequate supply in the blood in order for the body to manufacture thyroxine?

A. glucose
B. calcium
C. iodine   JODINE METABOLISM
D. fat

78. What could occur if all of the parathyroids are removed?   REGULATES CALCIUM LEVELS.

A. tetanus
B. ileus
C. thyroiditis
D. tetany

79. The principal hormone produced by the medulla of the adrenals is called   ADRENALIN

A. norepinephrine
B. ACTH
C. epinephrine
D. adrenosterone

80. The metabolic process produces

A. energy for the cell
B. new cells
C. protoplasm
D. tissue fluid

81. The largest of the endocrine glands is the

A. adrenal
B. parathyroid
C. pituitary
D. thyroid

82. The lungs are covered in a serous membranous sac called the

A. bronchial pleura
B. pulmonary pleura
C. visceral pleura
D. parietal pleura

83. Microscopic air sacs in the lung are called

A. alveoli
B. terminal bronchioles
C. bronchioles
D. bronchopulmonary segments

84. The smallest division of the bronchial tree is the

A. bronchial tubes
B. bronchi
C. alveoli
D. bronchioles

85. The passageway for foods and liquids into the digestive system, and for air into the respiratory system, is the

A. trachea
B. larynx
C. epiglottis
D. pharynx

86. The larynx is located between the

A. pharynx and the trachea
B. trachea and the bronchi
C. nasal cavity and the pharynx
D. pharynx and the bronchi

87. The vocal cords are located in the

A. larynx
B. pharynx
C. windpipe
D. trachea

88. Which structure has three divisions consisting of naso, oro, and laryngeal?

A. trachea
B. windpipe
C. larynx
D. pharnyx

89. The function of the trachea is to

A. conduct air into the larynx

B. serve as a pathway for food into the esophagus
C. serve as a resonating chamber for speech
D. conduct air to and from the lungs

90. When tears flow freely the nose runs, due to the

A. nasopharynx
B. sinus cavities
C. nasolacrimal duct
D. vascular plexus

91. The space between the vocal cords is called the

A. epiglottis
B. glottis
C. vocal fold
D. hilus

92. The nasal conchae are also known as the

A. turbinate bones
B. nasal septum
C. air passages
D. olfactory receptors

93. The nasal cavity is divided into two portions by the

A. concha
B. septum
C. ethmoid
D. vomer

94. The proximal phalanx refers to the bone of the finger that is

A. at the tip
B. in the middle
C. nearest the thumb
D. connected to the metacarpal

95. The bones of the palm of the hand are referred to as

A. phalanges
B. carpals
C. metacarpals
D. calcaneus

96. The muscles important in respiration are

A. trapezius
B. latissimus dorsi
C. pectoralis major
D. intercostal

97. The thick, fan-shaped muscle that lies on the anterior chest is the

A. latissimus dorsi
B. serratus anterior
C. pectoralis major
D. teres major

98. The triangular muscle of the shoulder which abducts the arm is the

A. biceps brachii
B. deltoid
C. triceps brachii
D. serratus anterior

99. Which of the abdominal muscles originates at the pubic bone and ends in the ribs?

A. rectus abdominis
B. transversus abdominis
C. external oblique
D. internal oblique

100. One of the principal muscles of the pelvic floor is the

A. sartorius
B. levator ani
C. internal oblique
D. rectus abdominis

101. The posterior thigh muscles are the

A. quadriceps femoris
B. iliopsoas
C. gastrocnemius
D. hamstrings

102. The largest muscle of the body, which acts to extend the leg at the hip, is the

A. quadriceps femoris
B. sartorius
C. gluteus maximus
D. adductor magnus

103. The gastrocnemius is the chief muscle of the

A. calf of the leg
B. stomach
C. stomach's greater curvature
D. thigh

104. A connective tissue band that holds bones together is called

A. cartilage
B. tendon
C. joint
D. ligament

105. The bone that forms the forehead, as well as the roof of the nasal cavity and the upper portion of the ocular orbits, is called

A. frontal bone
B. cranial bone
C. parietal bone
D. occipital bone

106. The two bones that form the side walls and the roof of the cranium are the

A. parietal bones
B. frontal bones
C. occipital bones
D. temporal bones

107. The sternocleidomastoid muscle is located

A. along the side of the neck
B. above and near the ear
C. under the tongue
D. in the back of the neck

108. The dorsal cavity includes the

A. thoracic cavity and the abdominal cavity
B. cranial cavity and the spinal cord
C. cranial cavity and thoracic cavity
D. cranial cavity and the abdominal cavity

109. All of the following are extrinsic eye muscles *except*

A. inferior rectus
B. superior rectus
C. orbicularis
D. superior oblique

110. When the vertebral column develops an abnormal lateral curve, the condition is called

A. kyphosis
B. lordosis
C. scoliosis
D. spondylosis

111. The medial bone of the forearm, which is located on the small-finger side of the hand, is called the

A. ulna
B. radius
C. humerus
D. fibula

112. The bone that is shaped like a butterfly and forms the anterior portion of the base of the cranium is the

A. temporal
B. sphenoid
C. ethmoid
D. parietal

113. The bone that forms the posterior portion of the skull is the

A. parietal
B. occipital
C. temporal
D. frontal

114. The lower jawbone is the

A. maxilla
B. mandible
C. mastoid
D. zygoma

115. The bone located in the neck between the mandible and the larynx, which supports the tongue and provides attachment for some of its muscles, is the

A. palatine bone
B. vomer
C. pterygoid hamulus
D. hyoid bone

116. The adult vertebral column has

A. 33 bones
B. 28 bones
C. 26 bones
D. 32 bones

7 cervical
12 THORACIC
5 LUMBAR
1 SACRAL
1 COCCYGEAL

117. The smallest vertebrae, forming a group of seven, are the

A. sacrum
B. cervical
C. thoracic
D. lumbar

118. Another name for the sternum is the

A. manubrium
B. gladiolus
C. costal cartilage
D. breastbone

119. The number of pairs of ribs is

A. 12
B. 10
C. 8
D. 7

120. Slender, rodlike bones which are located at the base of the neck and run horizontally are the

A. scapulae
B. shoulder blades
C. clavicles
D. sternum

121. The number of bones in the carpus is

A. 5
B. 8
C. 14
D. 16

122. Smooth muscle is found in all organs *except*

A. stomach

B. heart
C. gallbladder
D. intestines

123. The nucleus pulposus is the

A. cushioning mass within an intervertebral disk
B. result of a ruptured disk
C. outer layer of fibrocartilage within a disk
D. covering of the intervertebral disk

124. The principal muscle of mastication is the

A. masseter
B. sternocleidomastoid
C. platysma
D. orbicularis oris

125. The upper, flaring portion of hipbone is the

A. ischium
B. pubis
C. ilium
D. femoral head

126. Connective tissue that acts to cushion jolts and receives its nutrition from joint fluid is

A. synovia
B. ligament
C. tendon
D. cartilage

127. A large opening at the base of the skull through which the spinal cord passes is the

A. ossicle
B. hypoglossal canal
C. foramen ovale
D. foramen magnum

128. The bony basin of the body refers to the

A. hipbones
B. pelvis
C. acetabulum
D. ischium

129. The uppermost tarsal bone, which articulates with the fibula and the tibia, is the

A. calcaneus
B. talus TARSAL
C. cuboid
D. navicular

130. Fracture of the femur commonly occurs at the

A. head of the femur
B. lesser trochanter
C. neck of the femur
D. greater trochanter

131. The larger, weight-bearing bone of the lower leg is the

A. humerus
B. talus
C. fibula
D. tibia

132. The long, slender, twisted bone whose head articulates with the lateral aspect of the tibia is called the

A. fibula
B. talus
C. malleolus
D. calcaneus

133. The bone that fits into the acetabulum, forming a joint, is the

A. tibia
B. femur
C. fibula
D. patella

134. The kneecap is also called the

A. patella   (PATELLAR REALIGNMENT)
B. tibia
C. fibula
D. popliteal

135. A leg muscle located at the front of the leg which acts on the foot is the

A. rectus femoris
B. tibialis anterior
C. peroneus tertius
D. flexor digitorum longus

136. A fibrous membrane covering which supports and separates muscle is

A. muscle fiber
B. fascia
C. endomysium
D. epimysium

137. Keratin is

A. a tough protein substance in hair and nails
B. the pigment determining skin color
C. a hardened accumulation of ear wax
D. a water-soluble substance in the dermis

138. Another name for sebaceous glands is

A. sudoriferous glands
B. sweat glands
C. wax glands
D. oil glands

139. The membranes that line closed cavities within the body are called

A. mucous membranes
B. serous membranes
C. fascial membranes
D. skeletal membranes

140. The outermost layer of skin is the

A. epidermis
B. dermis
C. subcutaneous
D. corium

141. Insensible perspiration occurs when

A. drops of moisture are visible on the skin
B. evaporation of water vapor occurs with no moisture
C. the body is super-heated
D. the body is super-cooled

142. The longest bone in the body is the

A. femur
B. fibula
C. tibia
D. humerus

143. A rounded protuberance found at a point of articulation with another bone is called a

A. trochanter
B. trochlea
C. tubercle
D. condyle

144. A condition often occurring in old age, in which there is a generalized loss of bone substance due mainly to excessive bone resorption, is

A. osteoarthritis
B. osteomyelitis
C. osteoporosis
D. osteoblastoma

145. The epiphyses are the

A. ends of long bones
B. shafts of long bones
C. bone-forming cells
D. marrow-filled cavities within bone

146. The true skin, which has a framework of elastic connective tissue and is well supplied vascularly, is the

A. epidermis
B. vernix caseosa
C. dermis
D. subcutaneous

147. Cells responsible for forming new bone are
  A. fibroblasts
  B. osteoblasts
  C. red bone marrow
  D. yellow bone marrow

148. The shaft or middle part of a long bone is called the
  A. epiphysis
  B. diaphysis
  C. periosteum
  D. endosteum

149. The pigment granule that gives the skin its color is called
  A. melanoblast
  B. melanin
  C. melanoma
  D. melasma

150. The membrane that covers the bones is known as
  A. perichondrium
  B. synovia
  C. periosteum
  D. epithelium

periosteal elevator

151. The connective tissue that lies between organs and muscles, supporting blood vessels and nerves, is
  A. adipose tissue
  B. reticular tissue
  C. areolar tissue
  D. cartilage tissue

152. A broad, flat sheet of connective tissue that binds muscle firmly to bones or other muscle is
  A. aponeurosis
  B. myosin filament
  C. myofibrils
  D. sarcolemma

153. The membrane attached to the organs of the body is the
  A. parietal layer
  B. visceral layer
  C. superficial fascia
  D. deep fascia

154. The sensory receptor cells for the sense of smell are the
  A. odoriferous
  B. kakosmic
  C. parosmic
  D. olfactory

155. A transparent structure that permits the eye to focus rays to form an image on the retina is the
  A. sclera
  B. retina
  C. cornea
  D. lens

156. The purpose of the iris is to
  A. regulate the amount of light entering the eye
  B. protect the retina
  C. supply the choroid with nourishment
  D. receive images

157. The structure that is seen from the outside as the colored portion of the eye is the
  A. cornea
  B. pupil
  C. retina
  D. iris

158. The nerve that carries visual impulses to the brain is the
  A. ophthalmic nerve
  B. optic nerve
  C. oculomotor nerve
  D. trochlear nerve

159. The white outer layer of the eyeball is the
  A. conjunctiva
  B. sclera
  C. choroid
  D. retina

160. The posterior cavity of the eye contains
  A. cornea
  B. sclera
  C. vitreous humor
  D. aqueous humor

161. The portion of the ear that contains receptors for equilibrium is the
  A. semicircular canal
  B. cochlea
  C. mastoid antrum
  D. eustachian tube

162. The middle vascular layer of the eyeball is the
  A. sclera
  B. choroid
  C. retina
  D. cornea

163. The portion of the external ear visible at the sides of the head is the

A. auricle
B. external auditory canal
C. ossicle
D. vestibule

164. The structure that connects the middle ear and the throat, allowing the eardrum to vibrate freely, is the

A. membranous canal
B. external auditory canal
C. eustachian tube
D. semicircular canal

165. A term referring to a waxlike secretion in the external ear canal is

A. pinna
B. scala
C. aurium
D. cerumen

166. The conjunctiva is the

A. colored membrane of the eye
B. covering of the globe except for the cornea
C. gland that secretes tears
D. membrane lining the socket

167. The peripheral nervous system contains

A. cranial and spinal nerves
B. brain and spinal cord
C. peripheral nerves
D. spinal cord and spinal nerves

168. Sympathetic and parasympathetic are terms denoting the division of the

A. central nervous system
B. peripheral nervous system
C. autonomic nervous system
D. neuromuscular system

169. The number of pairs of spinal nerves is

A. 12
B. 28
C. 30
D. 31

170. The great sensory nerve of the face and head is the

A. trochlear
B. oculomotor
C. hypoglossal
D. trigeminal

171. The cranial nerve that contains special sense fibers for hearing as well as for balance is

A. II
B. V
C. VIII   8TH HEARING
D. XII

172. The pons   BRIDGE-LIKE PONDS.

A. controls the heart rate
B. forms a connection between the cerebellum and the rest of the nervous system
C. acts as a relay center for eye and ear reflexes
D. aids in voluntary muscle coordination

173. All thought takes place in the

A. midbrain
B. pons
C. cerebral cortex
D. cerebellum

174. The part of the brain responsible for maintenance of balance and muscle tone, as well as coordination of voluntary muscle, is the

A. cerebellum
B. cerebrum
C. midbrain
D. pons

175. The basic unit of the nervous system is the

A. neuron
B. nephron
C. dendrite
D. axon

176. Senses such as pain, touch, and temperature are interpreted in the

A. frontal lobe
B. parietal lobe   pain
C. temporal lobe
D. occipital lobe

177. The frontal, temporal, parietal, and occipital lobes are divisions of the

A. midbrain
B. interbrain
C. cerebellum
D. cerebrum

178. The area of the brain that controls the respiratory center is the

A. cerebellum
B. interbrain
C. pons
D. medulla oblongata   Rate + depth

179. The largest part of the brain is the

A. brainstem
B. cerebrum
C. diencephalon
D. cerebellum

180. The outermost covering of the brain and spinal cord is the

A. pia mater
B. dura mater
C. arachnoid
D. choroid

181. Cerebrospinal fluid circulates freely in the

A. subarachnoid space
B. arachnoid space
C. pia mater
D. subdural space

182. The brain contains four fluid-filled spaces called the

A. auricles
B. ventricles
C. fissures
D. sulci

183. Another name for the tympanic membrane is the

A. external auditory canal
B. eardrum
C. semicircular canal
D. hammer

184. The winding, cone-shaped tube of the inner ear is the

A. vestibule
B. semicircular canal
C. labyrinth
D. cochlea

185. The structure that serves as a boundary between the external auditory canal and the middle ear is the

A. bony labyrinth
B. ossicles
C. eustachian
D. tympanic membrane

186. The thick-walled structure that pumps blood out of the heart into the aorta is called the

A. right atrium
B. left atrium
C. right ventricle
D. left ventricle

187. The main function of hemoglobin is to

A. promote tissue healing
B. carry oxygen to the tissues
C. protect against hemorrhage
D. carry carbon dioxide to the tissues

188. The straw-colored portion of blood is called

A. fibrinogen
B. plasma
C. serum
D. lymphocyte

189. The volume percentage of red blood cells in whole blood is called

A. hemoglobin
B. CBC
C. hemolysis
D. hematocrit

190. The blood cell that functions mainly to destroy certain pathogens is

A. lymphocyte
B. leukocyte
C. erythrocyte
D. thrombocyte

191. From which source does the axillary artery receive its blood supply?

A. subclavian artery
B. innominate artery
C. brachial artery
D. brachiocephalic artery

192. A differential count provides an estimate of

A. the amount of hemoglobin
B. the volume percentage of red cells
C. the percentage of each type of white cell
D. electrolyte percentages

193. Mixing of incompatible bloods may result in

A. agglutination
B. infectious hepatitis
C. leukocytosis
D. hyperglycemia

194. The portion of blood responsible for the clotting process is

A. fibrinogen
B. lipids
C. platelets
D. plasma

195. Red blood cells are also known as

A. erythrocytes
B. leukocytes
C. lymphocytes
D. thrombocytes

196. Hemolysis can be defined as

A. overproduction of red blood cells
B. manufacture of red blood cells
C. breakdown of white blood cells
D. destruction of red blood cells

197. Erythrocytes are formed in the

A. lymph nodes
B. red bone marrow
C. yellow bone marrow
D. lymphoid tissue

198. In the normal adult the average number of leukocytes per cubic millimeter of circulating blood is

A. 1,000–4,000
B. 3,000–8,000
C. 5,000–10,000
D. 10,000–15,000

199. A large superficial vein in the lower extremity, which begins in the foot and extends up the medial side of the leg, the knee, and the thigh, is called the

A. femoral
B. greater saphenous
C. iliac
D. popliteal

200. The vein in the bend of the elbow that is commonly used as a site for venipuncture is the

A. subclavian vein
B. cephalic vein
C. median cubital vein   BETWEEN CEPHALIC AND SUBCLAVIAN VEIN
D. basilic vein

201. The artery at the back of the knee is the

A. popliteal   BEHIND KNEE
B. femoral
C. iliac
D. celiac

202. The superior and inferior mesenteric arteries supply which of the following organs?

A. stomach
B. intestines   MESENTARY
C. spleen
D. kidney

203. Which vein drains the veins of the chest wall and empties into the superior vena cava?

A. azygos
B. hepatic
C. cephalic
D. basilic

204. The palmer arch is a communication between the

A. two vertebral arteries
B. tibial arteries in the foot
C. branches of vessels in the large intestines
D. ulnar and radial arteries of the hand   PALM

205. The veins of the head and neck are drained by the

A. basilic vein
B. cephalic veins
C. azygos vein
D. jugular veins

206. Which arteries supply the heart?

A. pulmonary
B. aortic
C. coronary
D. common carotid

207. The atrioventricular (A-V) node causes

A. auricular relaxation
B. ventricular contraction   BY BUNDLE OF HIS AND PURKINJE FIBERS
C. ventricular dilation
D. auricular contraction

208. Why would an aspirated foreign body be more likely to enter the right bronchus rather than the left bronchus?

A. the right bronchus is more vertical, shorter, and wider than the left
B. the division of the right bronchus is wider
C. the right bronchus is longer
D. the left bronchus is not in line with the trachea

209. The spleen filters

A. antibodies
B. tissue fluid
C. lymph
D. blood

210. Circulation that is established through an anastomosis between two vessels supplying or draining two adjacent structures is called

A. portal circulation
B. collateral circulation
C. systemic circulation
D. pulmonary circulation

211. All of the following vessels branch off the aortic arch *except* the

A. left subclavian artery
B. brachiocephalic artery
C. left common carotid artery
D. coronary arteries

212. Which artery supplies the head and neck?

A. subclavian
B. carotid
C. brachiocephalic
D. aortic arch

213. The serous membrane that covers the heart is the

A. pericardium
B. myocardium
C. epicardium
D. endocardium

214. The circle of Willis is located

A. in the axillary region
B. posterior to the ear
C. at the base of the brain
D. at the base of the neck

215. The branch of the external iliac artery that is located in the thigh is called the

A. tibial artery
B. femoral artery   BECOMES THE POPLITEAL
C. popliteal artery
D. celiac artery

216. The descending aorta terminates at the level of the fourth lumbar vertebra, dividing into

A. two saphenous arteries
B. two femoral arteries
C. internal and external iliac arteries
D. two common iliac arteries

217. Which group of blood vessels concerns itself with eliminating carbon dioxide from the blood and replenishing its supply of oxygen?

A. capillaries
B. systemic veins
C. systemic arteries
D. pulmonary vessels

218. The chamber of the heart that pumps venous blood and sends it to the lungs is the

A. right atrium
B. left atrium
C. right ventricle
D. left ventricle

219. The thin-walled portion of the heart which receives the venous blood returning from the body is called the

A. right atrium
B. left atrium
C. right ventricle
D. left ventricle

220. The contractions of the heart are synchronized and regulated by the pacemaker of the heart, called the

A. sinoatrial node
B. atrioventricular node
C. atrioventricular bundle
D. Purkinje fibers

221. Tiny blood vessels that permeate and nourish tissue are called

A. veins
B. venules
C. arterioles
D. capillaries

222. The wall or partition dividing the heart into right and left sides is called the

A. semilunar valve
B. mitral valve
C. chordae tendineae
D. septum

223. Another name for the bicuspid valve is the

A. aortic
B. mitral
C. pulmonary
D. semilunar

224. Which heart valve closes at the time the right ventricle begins pumping, preventing blood from returning to the right atrium?

A. aortic semilunar
B. pulmonary semilunar
C. bicuspid
D. tricuspid

225. The inner lining of the heart, composed of smooth, delicate membrane, is called the

A. pericardium
B. endocardium
C. epicardium
D. myocardium

226. The spleen is located

A. in the left hypochondriac region
B. behind the liver
C. behind the left kidney
D. behind the right kidney

227. The thymus gland

A. manufactures thrombocytes
B. has no known function
C. plays a key role in immunity
D. produces hormones

228. The group of nodes which often enlarge during upper respiratory infections are the

A. tracheobronchial nodes
B. axillary nodes
C. cervical nodes
D. mesenteric nodes

229. All of the following are parts of the lymphatic system *except* the

A. thyroid
B. tonsils
C. spleen
D. thymus

230. The *s*-shaped bend in the lower colon is called the

A. hepatic flexure
B. splenic flexure
C. rectum
D. sigmoid

231. The main function of the large intestine is to

A. reabsorb water and electrolytes
B. digest food
C. absorb food nutrients
D. stimulate digestive juices

232. The terminal portion of the large intestine is the

A. sigmoid
B. rectum
C. anus
D. anal canal

233. The length of the large intestine is approximately

A. 5 ft
B. 12 ft
C. 18 ft
D. 20 ft

234. The double-layered structure that hangs from the lower border of the stomach, covering the intestines, is the

A. mesentery
B. lesser omentum
C. greater omentum
D. ligamentum

235. The first portion of the large intestine is the

A. sigmoid
B. cecum
C. colon
D. ileum

236. The appendix is attached to the

A. ascending colon

B. transverse colon
C. cecum
D. descending colon

237. The primary function of the gallbladder is

A. storage of bile
B. production of bile
C. digestion of fats
D. drainage of the liver

238. When the gallbladder contracts, bile is ejected into the

A. liver
B. duodenum
C. jejunum
D. pancreas

239. The area in the duodenum where the common bile duct and the pancreatic duct empty is called

A. the duct of Santorini
B. the ampulla of Vater
C. Wirsung's duct
D. an islet of Langerhans

240. The membrane lining the abdominal cavity and covering the surface of most of the abdominal organs is the

A. mesentery
B. greater omentum
C. lesser omentum
D. peritoneum

241. The common bile duct is the union of the

A. cystic duct and cystic artery
B. cystic duct and hepatic duct
C. cystic artery and hepatic duct
D. hepatic vein and cystic duct

242. The muscular folds of the stomach are the

A. rugae
B. follicles
C. vesicles
D. plica

243. The yellow tinge in the skin symptomatic of obstructive jaundice is due to the accumulation of what substance in the blood and tissue?

A. cholesterol
B. bile salts
C. enzymes
D. bilirubin

244. The head of the pancreas is located

A. in the curve of the duodenum
B. by the spleen
C. on the undersurface of the liver
D. in the curve of the descending colon

245. The portion of the small intestine that joins with the large intestine is called the

A. duodenum
B. jejunum
C. ilium
D. ileum

246. The valve at the junction of the small and large intestines is the

A. sphincter of Oddi
B. ileocecal sphincter
C. pyloric sphincter
D. duodenal sphincter

247. The portion of the small intestine that receives secretions from the pancreas and the liver is the

A. ileum
B. jejunum
C. duodenum
D. pylorus

248. The hormone released by the stimulation of certain stomach cells is

A. pepsinogen
B. gastrin
C. pepsin
D. amylase

249. The main components of gastric juice are

A. hydrochloric acid and enzymes
B. hydrochloric acid and gastrin
C. pepsin and gastrin
D. gastrin and enzymes

250. The portion of the stomach near the esophagus is the

A. cardiac
B. fundic
C. body
D. pyloric

251. A peritoneal fold encircling the greater part of the small intestines which connects the intestine to the posterior abdominal wall is the

A. lesser omentum
B. greater omentum
C. visceral peritoneum
D. mesentery

252. The balloonlike portion of the stomach that extends above the level of the junction with the esophagus is called the

A. pylorus
B. fundus
C. cardia
D. body

253. The muscle serving as a valve to prevent regurgitation of food from the intestine back into the stomach is known as the

A. sphincter of Oddi
B. ileocecal sphincter
C. cardiac sphincter
D. pyloric sphincter

254. How many divisions are there in the pharynx?

A. one
B. two
C. three
D. four

255. How do the exocrine glands work?

A. secrete products into ducts
B. secrete products into blood
C. secrete products into urine
D. digest fat

256. The digestive passageway that begins at the pharynx and terminates in the stomach is the

A. larynx
B. trachea
C. windpipe
D. esophagus

257. The point at which the esophagus penetrates the diaphragm is called the

A. hiatus
B. meatus
C. sphincter
D. fundus

258. The root or posterior tongue is anchored to the

A. maxillary bone
B. mandibular bone
C. hyoid bone
D. hard palate

259. The small, soft structure hanging from the free edge of the soft palate is the

A. frenulum
B. lingual tonsil
C. palatine tonsil
D. uvula

260. Pharyngeal tonsils is another name for

A. adenoids
B. palatine tonsils
C. uvula
D. masseters

261. When tonsils become infected and swollen they can interfere with breathing by blocking the

A. epiglottis
B. pharynx
C. trachea
D. eustachian tube

262. Chisel-shaped teeth whose sharp edges cut food are

A. cuspids
B. bicuspids
C. incisors
D. molars

263. Canines are also known as

A. molars
B. incisors
C. bicuspids
D. cuspids

264. Flat-surfaced teeth used for grinding hard particles are the

A. molars
B. deciduous teeth
C. incisors
D. cuspids

265. The canal or socket of a tooth is known as the

A. gingiva
B. alveolus
C. crown
D. roots

266. The parotid glands are located

A. under and in front of each ear
B. on the inner surface of the mandible
C. deep in the floor of the mouth
D. in the sublingual area

267. The salivary glands located under the tongue are the

A. subungual
B. sublingual
C. submaxillary
D. parotid

268. The liver has

A. two lobes
B. three lobes
C. four lobes
D. five lobes

269. The glomerulus is a

A. tiny coiled tube
B. tubelike extension into the renal pelvis
C. double-walled cup
D. cluster of capillaries

270. The tubes or cuplike extensions that project from the renal pelvis are called

A. glomeruli
B. convoluted tubules
C. Bowman's capsules
D. calyces

271. All are functions of the kidney *except*

A. acts as a reservoir for urine
B. is an organ of excretion
C. controls water balance
D. controls acid-base balance

272. Urine is transported along the ureters to the bladder by

A. gravity flow
B. contraction of the renal pelvis
C. peristaltic waves
D. muscle relaxation

273. The smooth, triangular area at the bottom of the bladder which contains three openings is called the

A. internal sphincter
B. urinary meatus
C. trigone
D. external os

274. Which of the following is *not* true of the male urethra?

A. is divided into three sections
B. is approximately 2.5 to 3 cm long
C. serves as a urine outlet
D. serves as a semen outlet

275. The kidneys are positioned

A. intraperitoneally
B. retroperitoneally
C. in front of the parietal peritoneum
D. in back of the visceral peritoneum

276. The functional unit of the kidney is the

A. glomerulus
B. nephron
C. medulla
D. cortex

277. Blood is supplied to the kidney by means of the renal artery, which arises from the

A. thoracic aorta
B. aortic arch
C. abdominal aorta
D. pulmonary artery

278. The inner layer of the kidney is known as the

A. medulla
B. glomerulus
C. nephron
D. cortex

279. The indentation in the kidney through which all structures must pass as they enter or leave the kidney is the

A. hilus
B. renal pelvis
C. renal capsule
D. cortex

280. The outer layer of the kidney is known as the

A. medulla
B. glomerulus
C. nephron
D. cortex

281. The portion of the male urethra that passes through the pelvic floor is called the

A. prostatic portion
B. cavernous portion
C. membranous portion
D. penile portion

282. Which of the following is a normal constituent of urine?

A. urea
B. albumin
C. glucose
D. ketone bodies

283. A severe toxic condition of the blood caused by failure of the kidneys to produce urine is

A. anuria
B. uremia
C. enuresis
D. anemia

284. Urinary retention is

A. lack of control of micturition
B. inability of the kidneys to produce urine
C. failure of ureters to carry urine to the bladder
D. failure to urinate

285. Lack of control over urination is called

A. retention
B. micturition
C. incontinence
D. suppression

286. Urine empties from the bladder through a tube called the

A. urethra
B. urinary meatus
C. urethral meatus
D. external urethral sphincter

287. The function of the bladder is to

A. produce urine
B. filter waste products
C. facilitate acid-base balance
D. act as a reservoir for urine

288. Fertilization occurs in the

A. fallopian tubes
B. uterus
C. ovary
D. gonads

289. The perineum is

A. a thin tissue stretching across the vagina
B. the region anterior to the clitoris
C. the lower portion of the uterus
D. the area between the vagina and the anus

290. Thin, highly vascular folds of tissue that contain sebaceous glands but no hair or sweat glands are the

A. labia minora
B. labia majora
C. vestibule
D. mons pubis

291. The small, sensitive structure of the female homologous to the male penis is the

A. hymen
B. clitoris
C. perineum
D. vestibule

292. The interior of the uterus is lined with highly vascular mucous membrane called

A. perimetrium
B. serosa
C. myometrium
D. endometrium

293. The space between the labia minora into which the vagina and urethra open is known as the

A. vestibule
B. vestibular bulb
C. vaginal orifice
D. urethral orifice

294. The dome-shaped part of the uterus above the uterine tubes is called the

A. body
B. corpus
C. fundus
D. cervix

295. Ova are swept into the fallopian tubes by small, fringelike extensions on the distal ends of the tubes called

A. ostium
B. fimbriae
C. oviducts
D. stroma

296. Ovulation occurs when the

A. ovum is fertilized
B. mature follicle ruptures
C. ovum is swept into the tube
D. egg implants in the endometrium

297. Glands lying deep in the perineal tissue that lubricate the vestibule and the vagina are the

A. bulbourethral glands
B. paraurethral glands
C. Bartholin's glands
D. lesser vestibular glands

298. What ligament attaches the ovaries to the pelvic wall?

A. mesovarian
B. ovarian
C. suspensory
D. broad

299. The supporting structure of the male reproductive system is the

A. inguinal canal
B. cremaster muscle
C. vas deferens
D. spermatic cord

300. The loose skin covering the glans penis like a sheath is called the

A. crura
B. prepuce
C. bulb
D. tunica albuginea

301. The distal end of the penis is slightly enlarged and is called the

A. glans penis
B. prepuce
C. foreskin
D. corpora cavernosa penis

302. The ejaculatory duct empties into the

A. prostate
B. penis
C. seminal vesicle
D. urethra

303. In a male, the structure surrounding the entrance to the urethra just below the urinary bladder is

A. Cowper's gland
B. the prostate gland
C. the bulbourethral gland
D. the seminal vesicle

304. The function of the seminal vesicles is to

A. nourish and protect sperm
B. store sperm
C. manufacture sperm
D. secrete sperm

305. The muscular tube that passes through the inguinal canal, enters the abdominal cavity, and ends behind the urinary bladder where it fuses with a seminal vesicle duct is called the

A. ejaculatory duct
B. spermatic cord
C. epididymis
D. vas deferens

306. The long, coiled tube in which sperm mature is the

A. vas deferens
B. epididymis
C. ejaculatory duct
D. seminal vesicle

C. MICROBIOLOGY

307. Who invented the first high-powered microscope?

A. Pasteur
B. Seuetos
C. Leeuwenhoek
D. Fracostorius

308. The first physician to practice aseptic technique was

A. Pasteur
B. Koch
C. Kircher
D. Lister

309. The smallest microbiologic organism is a

A. protozoan
B. protist
C. virus
D. bacterium

310. The process of weakening a vaccine is called

A. inactivation
B. agglutination
C. opsonization
D. attenuation

311. Bacteria in their sporative stage are

A. most resistant to destruction
B. least resistant to destruction
C. incapable of reproduction
D. incapable of function

312. Passage of fluid through a cell membrane is called

A. metosis
B. miosis
C. osmosis
D. symbiosis

313. Oxygen-dependent bacteria are said to be

A. anaerobic
B. bacillic
C. antibiotic
D. aerobic

314. The destruction of bacteria by white cells during the inflammatory process is called

A. symbiosis
B. mitosis
C. lymphocytosis
D. phagocytosis

315. Air droplets are the mode of transmission for all of the following *except*

A. colds
B. influenza
C. mumps
D. streptococcal infections

316. Vaccination against a disease provides

A. naturally acquired active immunity
B. artificially acquired active immunity
C. artificially acquired passive immunity
D. naturally acquired passive immunity

317. By which of the following methods of transmission would *Staphylococcus aureus* most likely be transmitted?

A. urine
B. feces
C. nose and mouth
D. sex organs

318. *Clostridium perfringens* causes gas gangrene and is classified as a/an

A. anaerobe
B. parasite
C. antigen
D. fungus

319. A foreign substance that stimulates the production of antibodies is a/an

A. antigen
B. endotoxin
C. exotoxin
D. resident flora

320. The clinical syndrome characterized by microbial invasion of the bloodstream is

A. superinfection
B. septicemia
C. cross-infection
D. cellulitis

321. Vaccines prepared from a localized infection are called

A. attenuated living vaccines
B. autogenous vaccines
C. toxoids
D. hyperimmune gamma globulins

322. Inflammatory exudate that is thick and yellow is termed

A. suppurative
B. fibrinous
C. serous
D. mucous

323. A relationship that benefits the organism at the expense of the host is called

A. mutualism
B. commensalism
C. parasitism
D. symbiosis

324. Bacteria reproduce most frequently by

A. binary fission
B. meiosis
C. spontaneous generation
D. sexual union

325. The ability of a pathogenic species to produce disease is known as its

A. virulence
B. pathogenicity
C. toxigenicity
D. infectivity

326. The transmitters of pathogenic organisms by mechanical or biologic means are called

A. vehicles
B. fomites
C. vectors
D. carriers

327. As pathogens are transmitted again and again, their virulence

A. decreases during an epidemic
B. increases during an epidemic
C. maintains endemic conditions
D. remains the same

328. The body's first line of defense against the invasion of pathogens is

A. the immune response
B. skin and mucous membrane linings
C. cellular and chemical responses
D. phagocytosis

329. Surgical maintenance of asepsis is the responsibility of the

A. OR supervisor
B. scrub person
C. circulating person
D. surgical team

330. Which access route is a major source of contamination in the OR environment?

A. parenteral
B. respiratory
C. alimentary
D. gastrointestinal

331. Spiral-shaped bacteria are identified as

A. bacilli
B. cocci
C. spirilla
D. spirochetes

332. One of the most important factors influencing wound healing is

A. nutrition of the patient
B. type of antibiotics
C. operative technique
D. housekeeping

333. Rubella is another name for

A. German measles
B. cold sores
C. chickenpox
D. measles

334. The basis for modern classification of organisms is the

A. Haeckel system
B. Linnaean system
C. Koch system
D. Kircher system

335. The simplest form of cell organization is the

A. protozoa
B. fungi yeast
C. fungi mold
D. bacteria

336. Herpes simplex is commonly called

A. cold sore
B. shingles
C. smallpox
D. chicken pox

337. All of the following descriptors refer to the inflammatory process *except*

A. heat
B. pain
C. vasoconstriction
D. edema

338. *Clostridium tetani* causes

A. gangrene
B. nosocomial infection
C. lockjaw
D. malaria

339. Fine, threadlike appendages that provide bacteria with motion are

A. pili
B. mesosomes
C. flagella
D. mitochondria

340. A valuable laboratory ally in identification of bacteria is

A. Gram stain
B. iodine stain
C. hang-drop stain
D. spore stain

341. Rod-shaped bacteria belong to the genus

A. *Spirillum*
B. *Bacillus*
C. *Coccus*
D. *Proteus*

342. A fulminating infection arising from necrotic tissue and spreading rapidly is

A. rabies
B. gas gangrene
C. pasteurellosis
D. tetanus

343. Rickettsiae are transmitted by

A. physical contact
B. airborne organisms
C. infected blood-sucking insects
D. infected animals

344. Which bacteria is commonly found in soil?

A. *Clostridium tetani*
B. *Trypanosoma brucci*
C. *Pediculus vestimenti*
D. *Yersina pestis*

345. Postulates to prove microbial origin were developed by

A. Henle
B. Koch
C. Lister
D. Pasteur

346. What bacteria causes rheumatic fever?

A. *Escherichia coli*
B. *Streptococcus*
C. *Pseudomonas*
D. *Staphylococcus*

347. A severe allergic reaction possibly resulting in death is called

A. arthus reaction
B. hypersensibility
C. anaphylactic shock
D. autoimmune disease

348. Fetal immunity is

A. naturally acquired passive
B. naturally acquired active
C. artificially acquired passive
D. artificially acquired active

349. What organism is responsible for a boil?

A. *Staphylococcus*

B. *Clostridium perfringens*
C. *Escherichia coli*
D. *Neisseria*

350. The organism most frequently found in burns is

A. *Clostridium perfringens*
B. *Pseudomonas aeruginosa*
C. *Clostridium tetani*
D. hemolytic streptococci

351. Scarlet fever is caused by

A. *Staphylococcus*
B. *Streptococcus*
C. *Escherichia coli*
D. *Pseudomonas*

352. Having origin within an organism is termed

A. endogeny
B. exogeny
C. endogamy
D. autogeny

353. One who is a "host of infection" but displays no symptoms is termed a

A. living reservoir
B. carrier
C. intermediary agent
D. transmitter

354. Diseases that are continually present in the community are considered

A. pandemic
B. epidemic
C. endemic
D. sporadic

355. Interferon is a/an

A. protein that kills viruses
B. protein that kills bacteria
C. chemically produced antiviral drug
D. antiviral vaccine

356. The "father of modern surgery" is

A. Pasteur
B. Halstead
C. Simpson
D. Lister

357. Gastroenteritis is caused by

A. *Shigella* organisms
B. *Enterobacterium*
C. *Isospora belli*
D. *Escherichia coli*

358. A bacterial pathogen most frequently invading damaged skin is

A. *Staphylococcus aureus*
B. *Clostridium tetani*
C. *Pseudomonas septica*
D. *Candida albicans*

359. Which type of wound would favor the development of gas gangrene?

A. moist
B. necrotic
C. dry
D. warm

360. An example of the autoimmune response is

A. asthma
B. tuberculosis
C. allergies
D. rheumatoid arthritis

361. Gas gangrene is caused by

A. *Fusobacterium*
B. *Clostridium tetani*
C. *Pseudomonas aeruginosa*
D. *Clostridium perfringens*

362. An enzyme produced by hemolytic streptococcus responsible for dissolving fibrin and delaying localization of a strep infection is

A. interferon
B. properdin
C. fibrinogen
D. fibrolysin

363. Venereal disease is generally transmitted by

A. direct person-to-person contact
B. blood contamination
C. indirect contamination
D. mucus-to-mucus contact

364. The bacteria highly resistant to sterilization and disinfection is

A. spores
B. fungus
C. gram-positive
D. pseudomonads

D. PHARMACOLOGY

365. A drug used to reverse hypotension is

A. Isuprel
B. Inderal
C. Pronestyl
D. Levophed

366. Demerol is a/an

A. analgesic
B. bronchial dilator
C. vasconstrictor
D. sedative

367. The Sengstaken–Blakemore tube is used for

A. esophageal hemorrhage
B. tonsillar hemorrhage
C. uterine hemorrhage
D. rectal hemorrhage

368. A specially treated form of surgical gauze that has a hemostatic effect when buried in tissue is

A. topical thrombin
B. Gelfoam
C. human fibrin foam
D. Oxycel

369. An anticoagulant given for its antagonistic effect on heparin is

A. dicumarol
B. Coumadin sodium
C. protamine sulfate
D. Dipaxin

370. A vitamin essential to the synthesis of prothrombin by the liver and a valuable hemostatic drug is

A. vitamin B
B. vitamin C
C. vitamin K
D. vitamin E

371. Which inhalation anesthetic agent is nonexplosive and nonflammable?

A. diethyl ether
B. penthrane
C. sodium pentothal
D. cyclopropane

372. Labor can be induced using

A. ergotrate
B. diazoxide
C. Pitocin
D. magnesium sulfate

373. Ergotamine, an oxytocic and vasoconstrictor, is used effectively in treating

A. ischemia
B. migraine headaches
C. cardiopulmonary disturbances
D. high blood pressure

374. In cataract surgery, which drug is given to dissolve the zonules that attach to the lens of the eye?

A. alpha-chymar
B. tetracaine
C. pilocarpine
D. cyclogyl

375. A miotic drug is

A. pilocarpine
B. homatropine
C. atropine
D. scopolamine

376. What topical anesthetic is used most frequently for preoperative ocular instillation?

A. lidocaine
B. tetracaine
C. cocaine
D. Dorsacaine

377. The drug added to a local ophthalmic anesthetic to increase diffusion is

A. alpha-chymotrypsin
B. hyaluronidase
C. epinephrine
D. Varidase

378. A radiopaque contrast media used in surgery is

A. methylene blue
B. gentian violet
C. renografin
D. cefazolin

379. Inflammation of the eye due to trauma is treated with

A. antibiotics
B. vasoconstrictors
C. steroids
D. ophthalmologic antiseptics

380. The action to be followed if a patient is experiencing a cardiac arrhythmia, specifically a ventricular fibrillation, would be to

A. start an intravenous
B. defibrillate
C. order blood to replace blood volume
D. administer intravenous lidocaine

381. An emergency drug useful in ventricular fibrillation or tachycardia is

A. Aramine
B. Xylocaine
C. Inderal
D. calcium chloride

382. An emergency drug that increases myocardial contractility is

A. calcium chloride
B. Levophed
C. Lasix
D. Isuprel

383. Dextran is used parenterally to

A. expand blood plasma volume
B. renourish vital tissue
C. carry oxygen through the system
D. decrease blood viscosity

384. Avitene is a/an

A. CNS depressant
B. anticoagulant
C. steroid hormone
D. hemostatic agent

385. The action of sodium bicarbonate in an advanced life support effort is to

A. stimulate heart muscle
B. strengthen and slow heart beat
C. reduce ventricular excitement
D. counteract metabolic acidosis

386. How many milliliters are in an ounce?

A. 10
B. 30
C. 75
D. 100

387. The last sensation to leave the patient during general anesthesia induction is

A. hearing
B. sight
C. feeling
D. smell

388. What drug treats an allergy?

A. antihistamines
B. beta blockers
C. antibiotic
D. anticoagulant

389. Keflin is a/an

A. antibiotic
B. steroid
C. mydriatic
D. diuretic

390. A solution used for eye irrigation is

A. phenylephrine HCl
B. normal saline
C. alphachymar
D. balanced salt solution

391. Pontocaine is

A. carbocaine
B. tetracaine HCl
C. marcaine
D. prilocaine HCl

392. One gram equals

A. 5 grains
B. 10 grains
C. 12 grains
D. 15 grains

393. An oxytocic drug used to stimulate uterine contraction is

A. Pitocin
B. Avitene
C. diazoxide
D. magnesium sulfate

394. Which drug can be added to saline for irrigation during a vascular procedure?

A. protamine
B. epinephrine
C. Sublimaze
D. heparin

395. A drug used to soothe and relieve anxiety is a/an

A. cholinergic
B. analgesic
C. sedative
D. narcotic

396. Which drug could be used to reverse the effect of muscle relaxants?

A. Narcan
B. protamine sulfate
C. Prostigmin
D. Valium

397. The basic unit of weight in the apothecaries' system of weights and measures is the

A. ounce
B. pound
C. grain
D. dram

398. Drugs used to reduce body temperature are called

A. antibiotics
B. antipyretics
C. antipruritics
D. antimetics

399. Steroids are used for

A. reduction of fluid in body
B. reduction of body's need for oxygen
C. reduction of tissue inflammation and swelling
D. reduction of uterine constriction and contraction

400. In which stage of anesthesia would anectine be mostly used?

A. induction
B. excitement
C. relaxation
D. danger

401. Soda lime is used in mask-inhalation anesthesia to

A. adjust anesthetic level
B. absorb carbon dioxide
C. absorb toxic elements
D. ventilate patient sufficiently

402. A method of anesthesia in which medication is injected into the subarachnoid space, affecting a portion of the spinal cord, is called a/an

A. Bier block
B. field block
C. nerve block
D. spinal block

403. A drug which reverses the action of morphine or other opiates is

A. Narcan
B. Pavulon
C. Prostigmin
D. protamine sulfate

404. A synthetic local anesthetic that is effective on mucous membrane and is used as a surface agent in ophthalmology is

A. Miochol
B. Zolyse
C. Dibucaine
D. tetracaine

405. Neuroleptanalgesia is the state resulting from the use of a combination of a

A. narcotic and an anticholinergic
B. narcotic and tranquilizer
C. tranquilizer and a hypnotic
D. narcotic and a hypnotic

406. All of the following are true of nitrous oxide *except*

A. induces poor relaxation
B. has a slow induction
C. is nonirritating
D. is good for minor surgery

407. A common complication of extubation is

A. hypotension
B. tachypnea
C. hypoxia
D. hypercapnia

408. The intraoperative diagnostic test that measures tissue perfusion is

A. blood volume
B. respiratory tidal volume
C. arterial blood gases
D. hematocrit

409. What is solu-Medrol?

A. antibiotic
B. myotic
C. mydriatic
D. anti-inflammatory

410. How many minims are there approximately in a cubic centimeter?

A. 10
B. 20
C. 30
D. 40

411. Xylocaine is used intravenously for

A. installation of local anesthesia
B. treatment of cardiac arrhythmias
C. diuretic action
D. restoration of blood volume

412. Nitrous oxide would be considered an ideal anesthetic agent if it were

A. nonexplosive
B. more potent
C. safer
D. odorless

413. Which nerves are first affected by local anesthesia?

A. vasomotor
B. sensory
C. motor
D. secretory

414. Another name for adrenalin is

A. ephedrine
B. epinephrine
C. lidocaine
D. Levophed

415. Which fact is *not* true of induced hypothermia?

A. it lowers body temperature
B. it reduces oxygen need of tissue
C. more anesthetic agent is needed
D. bleeding is decreased

416. The most common topical anesthetic agent used in ENT surgery is

A. xylocaine
B. procaine
C. cocaine
D. Surfacaine

417. The most frequently used barbiturate for intravenous anesthesia is

A. Ketamine
B. Anectine
C. Sublimaze
D. Pentothal

418. The total volume in a 30-cc syringe is

A. 1 ounce
B. 2 ounces
C. 3 ounces
D. 4 ounces

419. A drug used frequently for regional blocks is

A. tetracaine
B. novacaine
C. cocaine
D. Marcaine

420. All of the following statements are true of cyclopropane gas *except*

A. it is colorless
B. it is highly explosive
C. it produces a fair amount of relaxation
D. it produces an unpleasant induction

421. Approximately how many milliliters are there in a pint?

A. 250
B. 500
C. 750
D. 1000

422. Which method of inhalation anesthesia allows complete rebreathing of expired gases?

   A. open method
   B. semi-closed method
   C. closed method
   D. filtered method

423. The stage of anesthesia that begins with loss of consciousness is the

   A. first
   B. second
   C. third
   D. fourth

424. Morphine is used for

   A. pain
   B. hemorrhage
   C. vomiting
   D. spasm

425. An anticholinergic drug given preoperatively to inhibit mucus secretion is

   A. Demerol
   B. Talwin
   C. Atropine
   D. Narcan

426. Narcan is a/an

   A. narcotic
   B. vasoconstrictor
   C. anticholinergic
   D. narcotic antagonist

427. Anesthesia given in a combination of several agents to obtain optimum results is called

   A. regional anesthesia
   B. general anesthesia
   C. conduction anesthesia
   D. balanced anesthesia

428. What would be the indication for an epidural?

   A. anorectal, vaginal, perineal, and obstetric procedures
   B. lower intestinal procedures
   C. upper gastrointestinal procedures
   D. above the waist procedures

429. Miochol is a/an

   A. antihistamine
   B. blood thinner
   C. miotic
   D. anti-inflammatory

430. A vasoconstrictor which, when added to a local anesthetic agent, extends its life is

   A. ephedrine
   B. epinephrine
   C. aramine
   D. ethrane

E. WOUND HEALING

431. If the intestine is perforated or transected during surgery, abdominal sepsis may result from which bacteria?

   A. *Escherichia coli*
   B. *Proteus vulgaris*
   C. *Pseudomonas aeruginosa*
   D. *Staphylococcus aureus*

432. A surgeon known best for his "Principles of Tissue Handling" is

   A. Physick
   B. Hunter
   C. Halsted
   D. Pare

433. The burn classification that is characterized by dry, pearly white or charred-appearing surface is

   A. first
   B. second
   C. third
   D. fourth

434. Which vitamin enables the liver to produce clotting factors in the blood?

   A. C
   B. D
   C. E
   D. K

435. Clean cut wounds are called

   A. lacerated
   B. contused
   C. incised
   D. punctures

436. Inflammation is characterized by pain, redness, heat, swelling, and loss of function. The redness can be attributed to

   A. serum brought into the area
   B. constriction of capillaries
   C. vasodilation bringing more blood to the area
   D. heat from metabolic reaction

437. Removal of contaminated debris from a wound is called

A. decontamination
B. debridement
C. dehiscence
D. desiccation

438. The space caused by separation of wound edges is called

A. lag phase
B. evisceration
C. fibrous scarring
D. dead space

439. If tissue is approximated too tightly it can cause

A. ischemia
B. excessive scar tissue
C. keloids
D. adhesions

440. Tensile strength of a wound refers to

A. the suture strength
B. ability of tissue to resist rupture
C. wound contraction
D. tissue approximation

441. Dehiscence in a poor-risk surgical patient can be reduced by utilization of

A. interrupted sutures
B. heavier suture material
C. retention sutures
D. strong, tight dressing

442. The purpose of anticoagulant therapy is

A. to minimize the tendency of blood to clot in the vessels
B. to induce labor
C. to prevent inflammation
D. to prevent bacterial invasion

443. Overgrowth of granulation tissue is called

A. adhesions
B. proud flesh
C. keloid
D. scar tissue

444. The chief constituent of connective tissue is

A. fibrin
B. collagen
C. fibroplasia
D. serum protein

445. A blood protein that aids in clotting is

A. fibrinogen
B. prothrombin
C. fibrin
D. thrombin

446. A cicatrix is

A. an abscess
B. a scar
C. pus
D. a wound

447. Insufficient levels of oxygen in the circulation is called

A. hypotropia
B. hypoxemia
C. hypovolemia
D. ischemia

448. Good scar formation requires sufficient doses of

A. vitamin E
B. vitamin C
C. zinc
D. vitamin K

449. Keloids are

A. a form of abscess
B. an adhered serous membrane
C. a raised, thickened scar
D. a benign tumor

450. The formation of collagen in wound healing is interrupted by the medical administration of

A. anticoagulant therapy
B. steroid therapy
C. small doses of radiation
D. hormone therapy

451. A wound that is infected or one in which there is excessive loss of tissue heals by

A. primary intention
B. secondary intention
C. third intention
D. fourth intention

452. Following contaminated traumatic injury the patient must be preventatively treated for

A. hepatitis
B. gas gangrene
C. tetanus bacillus
D. bacteremia

453. Which type of wound healing requires debridement?

A. first
B. second
C. third
D. fourth

454. To promote healing, a surgical wound must have all of the following requisites *except*

A. suture closure of dead space

B. drains to remove fluid or air
C. a moderately tight dressing
D. tight sutures to create tension

455. Wound healing that employs a technique allowing the wound to heal from the bottom up is called

A. interrupted intention
B. first intention
C. second intention
D. third intention

F. GROSS ANATOMY

The Eye

Questions 456 through 466: Identify each numbered structure in the following diagram.

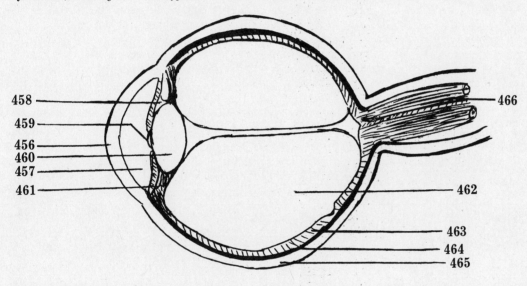

458
459
456
460
457
461

466

462

463
464
465

456. CORNEA
457. A. CHAMBER
458. P. CHAMBER
459. pupil
460. lens
461. iris
462. vitreous
463. retina
464. choroid
465. sclera
466. optic nerve

The Ear

Questions 467 through 475: Identify each numbered structure in the following diagram.

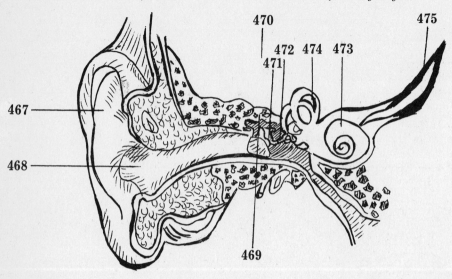

467. PINNA
468. Aud. Canal
469. tympanic mem.
470. malleous
471. incus
472. stapes
473. cochlea
474. semicircular
475. auditory nerve

The Heart

Questions 476 through 485: Identify each numbered structure in the following diagram.

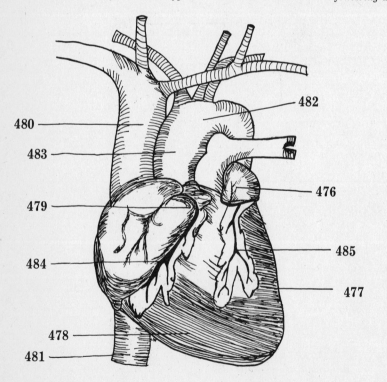

476. L. AURICLE
477. L. VENTRICLE
478. R. VENTRICLE
479. R. AURICLE
480. S. VENA CAVA
481. I. vena cava
482. Arch of Aorta
483. ascending Aorta
484. R. coronary Art
485. L coronary Art

The Respiratory System

Questions 486 through 497: Identify each numbered structure in the following diagram.

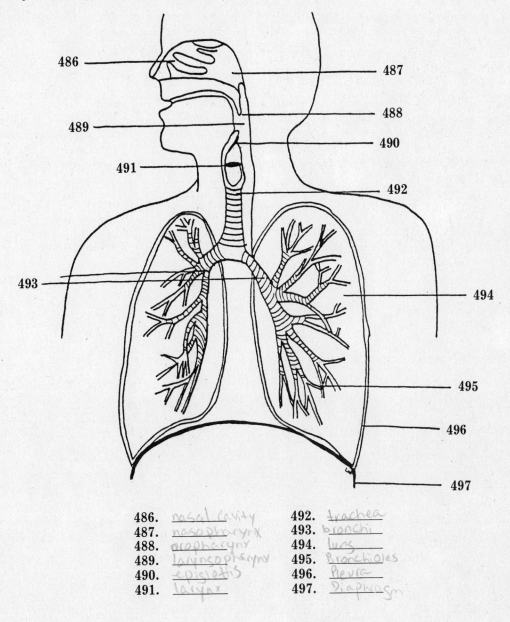

486. nasal cavity
487. nasopharynx
488. oropharynx
489. laryngopharynx
490. epiglottis
491. larynx

492. trachea
493. bronchi
494. lung
495. bronchioles
496. pleura
497. diaphragm

The Urinary System

Questions 498 through 502: Identify each numbered structure in the following diagram.

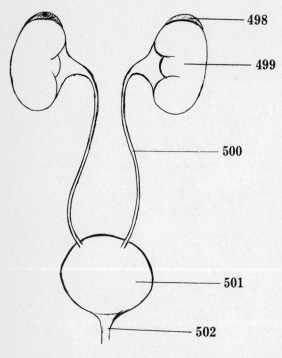

498.
499.
500.
501.
502.

498. Adrenal gland
499. kidney
500. ureter
501. bladder
502. urethra

The Kidney

Questions 503 through 510: Identify each numbered structure in the following diagram.

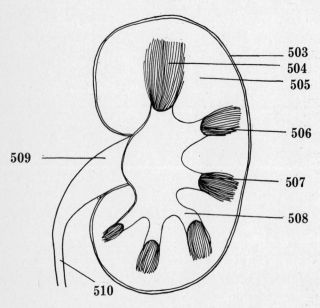

503.
504.
505.
506.
507.
508.
509.
510.

503. fibrous capsule
504. medulla
505. cortex
506. pyramid
507. papilla
508. calyx
509. renal pelvis
510. ureter

The Brain

Questions 511 through 517: Identify each numbered structure in the following diagram.

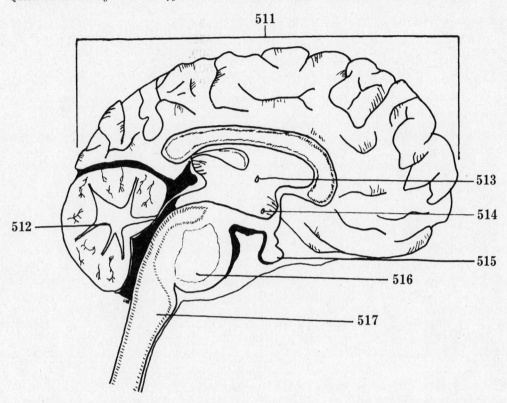

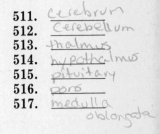

511. cerebrum
512. cerebellum
513. thalmus
514. hypothalmus
515. pituitary
516. pons
517. medulla oblongata

The Skull

Questions 518 through 527: Identify each numbered structure in the following diagram.

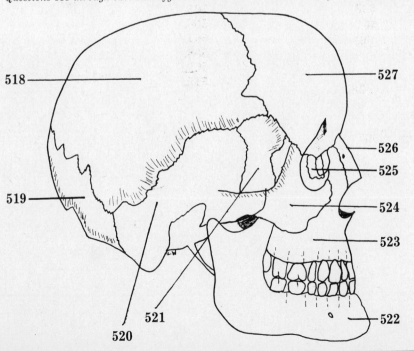

518. parietal
519. occipital
520. temporal
521. sphenoid
522. mandible
523. maxilla
524. zygomatic arch
525. lacrimal bone
526. nasal bone
527. fronta

Forms of Bacteria

Questions 528 through 534: Identify each numbered structure in the following diagram.

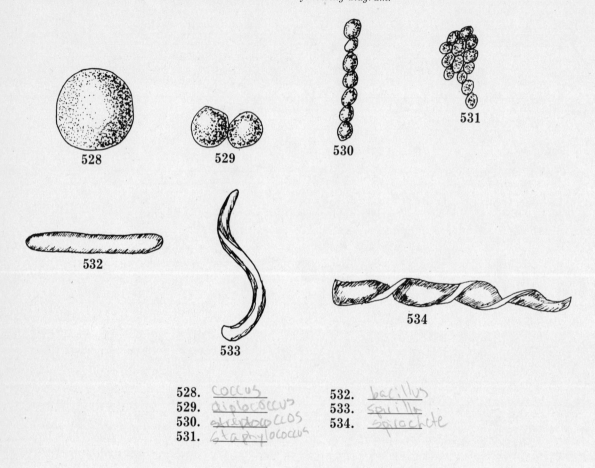

528.   coccus   532.   bacillus
529.   diplococcus   533.   spirilla
530.   streptococcus   534.   spirochete
531.   staphylococcus

Answers and Explanations

A. TERMINOLOGY

1. **(B)** The root word *glosso* denotes the tongue, as in glossitis (inflammation of the tongue). Hypoglossal means under the tongue. *(36:689)*

2. **(B)** *Choledochal* refers to the common bile duct; *itis* means inflammation of. Choledochitis thus is inflammation of the common bile duct. *(36:318)*

3. **(D)** Acute means sharp, severe, and having a rapid onset. It is exhibited by severe symptoms and a short course. Chronic means long, drawn out or a disease of slow progress. *(36:34, 329)*

4. **(C)** The suffix *cyte* denotes a cell. The root to which it is attached designates the type of cell. An example is erythrocyte (red blood cell). *(3:53)*

5. **(D)** The submental region is located below the chin. *Mentum* means chin. *Sub* means below or under. *(3:52)*

6. **(B)** The root word *meso* means middle or mid. Mesoderm means middle layer of the skin. Mesocarpal means middle of the wrist. *(3:217)*

7. **(C)** The prefix *pseudo* means false or spurious. Pseudocirrhosis means apparently like cirrhosis. Pseudocyesis means false pregnancy. (Cyesis means pregnancy.) *(36:1399)*

8. **(B)** The root word *adeno* means gland. Adenitis means gland inflammation. Adenocarcinoma is a malignant adenoma arising from a glandular organ. *(36:36)*

9. **(D)** PRN stands for pro re nata. This means according to circumstances. It also means as necessary. *(36:1390)*

10. **(C)** NPO means nada per os (opening), or nothing by mouth. A patient is NPO prior to surgery, which means that he or she receives no food or drink for at least 8 hours prior to the time of the procedure. *(36:1933)*

11. **(B)** The term distal refers to an area away from the point of origin. It means farthest away from the medial line or trunk. The hand is distal to the elbow. *(3:50)*

12. **(A)** Proximal is nearest to the point of attachment, or point of reference. It is the opposite of distal. *(36:1397)*

13. **(C)** The addition of *ectomy* to the term representing any anatomic organ denotes surgical removal of the organ. Tonsillectomy is removal of the tonsils. Splenectomy is removal of the spleen. *(3:191)*

14. **(A)** The symbol gtt means a drop. Gtts means drops. *(36:1935)*

15. **(A)** *Endo* means within. Endocervical means within the cervix. Endocardium means within the heart. *(3:9)*

16. **(A)** The appendix is located at the base of the cecum in the right lower quadrant. It is a wormlike process. It is also called the veriform appendix. *(36:121)*

17. **(A)** Abduction means movement away from the median plane. Frequently in surgery, the surgeon may request that a limb be abducted which means moved away from the body. *(36:5)*

18. **(C)** CO_2 represents the gaseous compound carbon dioxide. Carbon dioxide is a colorless gas and it is heavier than air. *(36:266)*

19. (B) Oncology is the study of scientific control over neoplastic growths. It concerns the etiology, diagnosis, treatment, and rehabilitation of cancer patients.

(2:472)

20. (B) *Algia* is the suffix signifying pain. Neuralgia is a painful nerve. Arthralgia is pain in a joint. *(36:57)*

21. (B) *Oma* is a suffix that denotes a tumor or neoplasm. Hepatoma means tumor of the liver. Fibroma is a fibrous tumor. *(2:472))*

22. (D) The suffix *oscopy* means viewing of organs. Cystoscopy is an examination of the interior of the urinary bladder. Bronchoscopy is an examination of the bronchi through a lighted bronchoscope. *(2:356)*

23. (A) A cubic centimeter (cc) is equivalent to a milliliter. Milliliter is used when referring to liquid volume. Cubic centimeter is used when referring to volume such as that of a gas. *(36:1055)*

24. (B) The term stenosis means constriction or narrowing of a passage. It is synonymous with stricture. Pyloric stenosis is an obstruction of the pyloric orifice. *(36:1623)*

25. (B) The suffix *lysis* indicates reduction or relief of a condition. It also means dissolution or decomposition of. Hemolysis is the destruction of red blood cells. *(36:990)*

26. (B) The root word *brady* means slow. Bradycardia is a slow heart beat. Bradypnea is abnormally slow breathing. *(2:27; 36:225)*

27. (A) A milliliter (ml) is equal to one one-thousandth (1/1000) of a liter. A milliliter is used when referring to liquid volume. *(36:1055)*

28. (B) The prefix *contra* means against or opposite. Contraindicate means against indication. Contraception is a process, device, or method that prevents conception. *(36:376)*

29. (A) Pelvic inflammatory disease (PID) is a collective term for any extensive bacterial infection of the pelvic organs. It especially refers to the uterus, tubes, and ovaries. Salpingitis is an infection in the tubes. *(38:726)*

30. (C) A polyp is a growth extending outward from a mucous membrane. Polyps are usually benign, but may be malignant. A tumor with a pedicle. *(36:1344)*

31. (B) Dysuria is painful or difficult urination. It is symptomatic of many conditions. Cystitis or a urinary tract infection can cause dysuria. *(36:508)*

32. (C) A cystocele is a herniation of the urinary bladder into the vagina. Frequently these are due to trauma following childbirth. A synonym is vesicocele. *(3:218; 36:414)*

33. (C) Uremia is a disturbed kidney function in which urinary constituents are found in the blood, producing a toxic condition. Substances normally excreted are retained in the blood. *(3:218)*

34. (C) Arteriosclerosis is hardening of the walls of arterioles, with resultant loss of elasticity and contractility. The walls can also thicken. This can cause compromised circulation. *(3:140)*

35. (D) Splenomegaly means enlargement of the spleen. Massive splenomegaly may require splenectomy. Enlargement may be associated with hemolytic disease of the blood. *(3:139)*

36. (C) Peristalsis is wormlike movements by which the alimentary canal propels its contents. The wavelike movements are involuntary and consist of simultaneous relaxations and contractions. *(36:1268; 3:185)*

37. (A) Profunda refers to anything that is deep-seated. This term is often applied to blood vessels deeply located. *(36:1386)*

38. (A) Increase in the size of an organ or structure by virtue of an increase in cell size is called hypertrophy. An increase due to actual cell number is hyperplasia. This does not involve tumor formation. *(36:805)*

39. (B) The prefix *ab* means away from. Abducting means leading away from. *Ad* means toward. Adducting means leading toward. *(36:1, 34)*

40. (B) The root word *edema* indicates swelling. Myoedema means muscle swelling. Lymphedema means lymphatic swelling. Edematous pertains to or is effected with edema. *(3:22)*

41. (D) The suffix *oid* expresses resemblance. Epidermoid means resembling epidermis. A dermoid cyst is a cyst containing hair, teeth, or skin. *(3:13)*

42. (B) An osteochondroma is a tumor containing bone and cartilage. *(3:74)*

43. (A) The term flaccid is applied to muscles with less than normal tone which may be a result of damage or disease of the nerve that conducts a constant flow of impulses to the muscle. If the muscle does not receive impulses for an extended period of time, it may progress from flaccidity to atrophy. *(38:214)*

44. **(C)** Atrophy is a state of wasting away. Individual muscle cells decrease in size. Bedridden people or those with casts experience atrophy because the flow of impulses to the inactive muscle is greatly reduced. If nerve supply is cut, it will undergo complete atrophy.   *(38:214)*

45. **(B)** The root word *lingua* indicates tongue. Lingual means pertaining to the tongue. Bilingual refers to two geographic tongues.   *(3:15)*

46. **(C)** The root word *homo* represents same or like. Homogeneous is of the same species or type. Homosexual is one sexually attracted to the same sex. *Hema, hemato,* and *haemo* are all terms referring to blood.   *(3:28)*

47. **(B)** A fossa is a basinlike depression in a bone. It is a furrow or shallow depression. The iliac fossa is a concavity on the iliac bone.   *(3:162)*

48. **(C)** *Litho* or *lith* are prefixes pertaining to a stone or calculus. Lithocystotomy is an incision of the bladder to remove a stone. Cholelithiasis is the presence of a stone in the gallbladder.   *(36:318, 968)*

49. **(B)** An inch is equal to 2.54 cm. To convert inches to centimeters multiply by 2.54. To convert centimeters to inches multiply by 0.3937.   *(36:295)*

50. **(A)** The prefix *de* means away from. Decompensation means failure of compensation. It also means down as in decompression, removal of pressure.   *(36:422)*

51. **(B)** Hypoxia is the reduction in oxygen supply to the cells. Deficiency of oxygen. Decreased concentration of oxygen in the inspired air.   *(38:576; 36:814)*

52. **(D)** The directional term dorsal indicates the area near or on the back. Indicating a position toward a rear part. Opposite or ventral.   *(36:487)*

53. **(C)** Necrosis indicates a death of a section of tissue or bone surrounded by healthy tissue. The dead bone is called sequestrum. Dead tissue is called slough.   *(36:1103)*

54. **(C)** The prefix *supra* means above or beyond. Suprascapular means on the upper scapula. Supralumbar is above lumbar. Suprapubic is above the pubic arch.   *(36:1659)*

55. **(A)** The prefix *a* or *an* means without or lack of. Apathy means lack of emotion. Apnea means lack of respiration. Anemic means without red blood cells.   *(3:8)*

56. **(B)** Dysmenorrhea refers to pain in association with menstruation. It is a frequent gynecologic disorder.

Dys refers to difficult, *men* to month, and *rhein* to flow.   *(36:505)*

57. **(B)** The nipple contains erectile tissue. It is surrounded by a pigmented area called the areola. The areola may be darker in those who have borne children.   *(36:1128)*

58. **(C)** The gingiva is the gum. It is the tissue surrounding the necks of the teeth and covering the alveolar processes of the maxilla and the mandible.   *(36:679)*

59. **(D)** The formation of a blood clot inside a vessel, partially or completely closing it, is called a thrombosis. The clot itself is called a thrombus. It may damage tissue by cutting off its blood supply.   *(38:446)*

60. **(D)** Bradycardia indicates a slow heart rate or pulse rate. The average pulse rate is between 70 and 90 beats per minute. In bradycardia, it is under 50 beats per minute.   *(38:492)*

61. **(A)** The term tachycardia means rapid heart or pulse rate. The average pulse rate is between 70 and 90 beats per minute. In tachycardia, it is over 100 beats per minute.   *(38:492)*

62. **(D)** Referred pain is pain seeming to rise in an area other than its origin. An example would be in appendicitis as often the pain seems to occur in areas other than that of the appendix location.   *(36:1208)*

63. **(A)** Intractable pain is pain that cannot be easily relieved. This pain often occurs in certain neoplastic invasions.   *(36:1207)*

64. **(D)** A cyst is a closed sac or pouch with a definite wall. It can contain fluid, semifluid, or solid material. It is usually an abnormal structure resulting from developmental anomalies, obstruction of ducts, or from parasitic infections.   *(36:412)*

65. **(C)** An ulcer is an open sore or lesion of the skin or mucous membrane accompanied by sloughing of inflamed necrotic tissue. It is sometimes accompanied by pus formation.   *(36:1797)*

66. **(B)** A fibroma is a benign, fibrous, encapsulated connective tissue tumor, irregular in shape, slow in growth, and has a firm consistency. A glioma, a Ewing's tumor, and sarcomas are all cancerous tumors.   *(36:581, 618, 686, 1519)*

67. **(C)** Muscular hypertrophy is an increase in the size of an organ or structure which does not involve tumor formation. It is restricted to an increase in size or bulk not resulting from an increase in the number of cells or tissue elements.   *(36:805)*

68. **(B)** A fissure is a groove or natural division. It is an ulcer or cracklike sore on the margin of the anus. A fistula is an abnormal tubelike passageway from a normal cavity or tube to a free surface or to another cavity. *(36:622–623)*

69. **(C)** Evulsion means tearing away of a part or new growth. It is the same as avulsion. An avulsion fracture is defined as tearing of a piece of bone away from the main bone by the force of muscular contraction. *(36:163, 581, 644)*

70. **(D)** The lacrimal gland is another name for tear sac. (Greek: *dakyron,* tear). (Greek: *ade,* gland). It can become inflamed and if prolonged can cause obstruction of the nasolacrimal duct. *(36:419)*

B. ANATOMY AND PHYSIOLOGY

71. **(B)** The thyroid gland produces thyroxine. This regulates metabolism for the production of heat and energy in body tissue. The primary function is iodine metabolism. *(27:214)*

72. **(B)** The adrenal glands are located above each kidney. They are glands of internal secretion. They are also called the suprarenals. *(36:40)*

73. **(C)** The parathyroids are four tiny epithelial bodies located behind the thyroid gland. They are embedded in its capsule. They secrete parathormone which regulates calcium metabolism. *(36:1233)*

74. **(D)** Islets of Langerhans are dispersed throughout the pancreas. Glucagon and insulin are the endocrine secretions concerned with regulation of blood sugar levels. *(38:421)*

75. **(C)** The anterior pituitary gland produces somatotropic hormone (growth hormone), gonadotropic hormones (controlling development of the reproductive system), thyrotropic hormone (stimulates the thyroid), adrenocorticotropic hormone (stimulates the cortex of the adrenal gland), and lactogenic hormone (stimulates milk production in the female). *(38:407–412)*

76. **(B)** The pituitary or master gland is a small gland about the size of a cherry. It is located in the brain. Its hormones are also called hypophysis. *(38:406)*

77. **(C)** In order for thyroxine to be manufactured, there must be an adequate supply of iodine in the blood. Thyroxine regulates metabolism, growth and development, and the activity of the nervous system. *(38:803)*

78. **(D)** Tetany is a nervous affliction characterized by intermittent muscular twitching and spasms involving the extremities and also convulsions. It can occur by the inadvertent operative removal of the parathyroids during thyroidectomy. The hormone parathormone produced by the parathyroids regulates the amount of calcium in the blood. *(36:252, 1233, 1714)*

79. **(C)** The principle hormone produced by the medulla of the adrenal gland is adrenaline or epinephrine. It works during emergency situations, causing the blood pressure to rise and the heartbeat to increase. *(27:215)*

80. **(A)** The chain of chemical reactions by which food is transformed for use by the cells is given the broad term metabolism. The metabolic process produces energy, which is the capacity for action by the cell. *(27:18)*

81. **(D)** The thyroid gland, located in the neck, is the largest endocrine gland. It has a right and left lateral lobe on either side of the trachea. It is connected by an isthmus located in front of the trachea just below the cricoid cartilage. *(38:803)*

82. **(C)** Each lung is enveloped in a sac of serous membrane called the pleura. The chest cavity is lined with the parietal pleura. The lung covering is called the visceral pleura. *(27:174)*

83. **(A)** At the end of each of the smallest bronchioles is a cluster of air sacs, alveoli. They resemble a bunch of grapes. They share a common opening. *(27:174)*

84. **(D)** Each bronchial tube subdivides, forming progressively smaller divisions. The smallest division is called a bronchiole. *(27:174)*

85. **(D)** The muscular pharynx serves as a passageway for food and liquids into the digestive tract. It also is the path for air into the respiratory system. The throat runs from the nares and runs partway down the neck where it opens into the esophagus (posterior) and the larynx (anterior). *(38:543–545)*

86. **(A)** The larynx is located between the pharynx and the trachea or windpipe. It is also called the voicebox. It is composed of muscle and cartilage. *(38:545, 547)*

87. **(A)** The vocal cords lie in the upper end of the larynx. They are responsible for voice production. *(38:546)*

88. **(D)** The pharynx has three divisions. The upper is behind the nasal cavity (nasopharynx). The middle section is behind the mouth (oropharynx). The lowest section is called the laryngeal pharynx. *(38:543–544)*

89. **(D)** The windpipe or trachea conducts air to and from the lungs. It is a tubular passageway located anterior to the esophagus. It further divides into the right and left bronchi.   *(38:547)*

90. **(C)** The nasolacrimal duct is a small duct in the nasal cavity. It communicates directly with the tear-producing glands.   *(27:111, 173)*

91. **(B)** The space between the two vocal folds in the larynx is called the glottis. If anything but air passes into the larynx, a cough reflex attempts to expel the material.   *(38:545)*

92. **(A)** The nasal conchae are also known as the turbinate bones. They curl out from the lateral walls of the nasal cavity on each side. They divide the cavity into three distinct air passageways.   *(21:569)*

93. **(B)** The nasal cavity is a hollow behind the nose. It is divided into right and left portions by the nasal septum. The anterior septum is made of cartilage.   *(38:542)*

94. **(D)** The phalanges are the bones forming the framework of the fingers. Each of these bones is called a phalanx. Exact identification may be made by using the word "distal" for the tips, "middle" for the next group, and "proximal" for those connected with the metacarpal bones.   *(27:61)*

95. **(C)** The metacarpal bones form the palm of the hand. There are five on each side. Their distal ends form the knuckles.   *(27:61)*

96. **(D)** The intercostal muscles are inserted in the spaces between the ribs. These are particularly important in respiration. They serve to enlarge the thoracic cavity upon inspiration.   *(27:77)*

97. **(C)** The pectoralis major is a thick, fan-shaped muscle located in the upper chest. Its fibers extend from the center of the thorax through the armpits to the humerus.   *(21:275)*

98. **(B)** The deltoid is a thick, triangular muscle that covers the shoulder joint. It is responsible for the roundness of the shoulder. It acts to abduct the arm.   *(34:194)*

99. **(A)** On the anterior portion of the abdominal wall, the rectus abdominis forms a straplike mass of muscle. It runs from the pubic bone at the floor of the abdominal cavity straight up to the xiphoid process of the sternum and the lower margins of the rib cage.   *(34:185–190)*

100. **(B)** The pelvic floor, or perineum, has its own form of diaphragm shaped somewhat like a shallow dish. One of the principle muscles of this pelvic diaphragm is the levator ani, which acts on the rectum and aids in defecation.   *(27:77)*

101. **(D)** The posterior thigh muscles are called hamstrings. Their tendons can be felt behind the knee on both sides. One of the tendons form the medial and lateral boundaries of the popliteal space.   *(27:77)*

102. **(C)** The gluteus maximus, in the buttocks, is the largest muscle in the body. It is a powerful extension of the thigh. It rotates the lower extremity laterally. *Glutos* means buttocks. *Maximus* means large.   *(34:203)*

103. **(A)** The gastronemius is the chief muscle of the calf of the leg. It is a large muscle on the posterior part of the leg. It extends the foot and helps to flex the knee upon the thigh.   *(36:666)*

104. **(D)** A ligament is a band or sheet of strong fibrous tissue connecting the articular ends of bones. It serves to bind them together and facilitate or limit motion. It is a cordlike structure.   *(36:954)*

105. **(A)** The frontal bone forms the framework for the forehead. The roof between the eyeballs and the frontal parts of the cerebrum contains airspaces and sinuses.   *(27:53)*

106. **(A)** One parietal bone is located on each side of the skull just posterior to the frontal bone. They form the bulging sides and the roof of the cranium.   *(21:196)*

107. **(A)** The sternocleidomastoid muscle extends along the side of the neck. It is sometimes referred to as the sternomastoid. It arises from the sternum and the inner part of the clavicle.   *(36:1626)*

108. **(B)** Within the dorsal cavity are located the brain and the spinal cord. It is located near the posterior surface of the body. Pertaining to the back or rear.   *(38:13)*

109. **(C)** Of the six pairs of extrinsic muscles of the eyes, four are straight muscles. They are named according to their position relative to the eyeball and the action that they produce: medial, lateral, superior, and inferior rectus. The remaining two, the superior and the inferior oblique, have a slanting arrangement.   *(34:177)*

110. **(C)** The vertebral column can develop an abnormal curve laterally. At the same time, the thoracic and abdominal organs may be displaced or compressed. This condition is called scoliosis.   *(27:63)*

111. **(A)** The forearm is the ulna. It is on the same side as the little finger. On the proximal end is the olecranon process which forms the prominence of the elbow.
(38:164–166)

112. **(B)** The sphenoid bone is a large wedge-shaped bone at the base of the skull. It lies between the occipital and ethmoid in the front, and between the parietal and temporal bones on the side.
(36:1596)

113. **(B)** The occipital bone forms the posterior part and a good portion of the base of the cranium. It is the bone in the lower part of the skull between the parietal and the temporal bones.
(36:1151)

114. **(B)** The mandible is the lower jawbone. It is the only movable bone in the skull. It is horseshoe shaped.
(36:1003)

115. **(D)** The hyoid bone is located in the neck between the mandible and the larynx. It supports the tongue and provides an attachment for its muscles. It does not articulate with any other bone.
(38:151)

116. **(C)** In an infant there are 33 separate bones in the vertebral column. Five of these bones eventually fuse to form the sacrum, and four others join to become the coccyx. As a result an adult vertebral column has 26 parts.
(38:151)

117. **(B)** Seven cervical vertebrae comprise the bony axis of the neck. Although these are the smallest of the vertebrae, their osseous tissues are denser than those of any other.
(38:155)

118. **(D)** The sternum is located along the midline in the anterior portion of the thoracic cage. It is also called the breastbone. It is flat, narrow, and about 6 inches long.
(38:158)

119. **(A)** Regardless of age, each person usually has 12 pairs of ribs, one pair attached to each of the 12 thoracic vertebrae. Each rib articulates posteriorly with its corresponding thoracic vertebrae.
(38:158)

120. **(C)** The clavicles are slender, rodlike bones with elongated s-shapes. They are located at the base of the neck and run horizontally between the sternum and the shoulders. Another name is collarbone.
(38:164)

121. **(B)** The carpus, or wrist, consists of eight small bones united to each other by ligaments. Four bones are in each row. There are two transverse rows.
(38:166)

122. **(B)** Smooth muscle tissue occurs in layers within the walls of hollow visceral organs and functions automatically without conscious effort. For this reason it is sometimes called involuntary.
(21:118)

123. **(A)** Each disk is composed of a tough outer layer of fibrocartilage (annulus fibrosus) and an elastic central mass (nucleus pulposus). This structure is soft and pulpy.
(38:157)

124. **(A)** There are four pairs of muscles for chewing, all of which insert on the mandible and move it. The largest are the temporal and the masseter muscles.
(38:232)

125. **(C)** The upper, flaring portion or prominence of the hipbone is the ilium. Its superior border is the iliac crest. The internal surface is the iliac fossa.
(34:127)

126. **(D)** Cartilage, a type of connective tissue, is relatively hard, with a smooth surface and no direct blood supply. Its nutrition is derived from joint fluid and its main action is to cushion jolts and bumps.
(38:97)

127. **(D)** The foramen magnum is a large hole in the inferior part of the bone (occipital) through which the medulla oblongata and its membranes, the accessory nerve (XI), and the vertebral and spinal arteries pass. Opening of the occipital bone through which passes the spinal cord from the brain.
(38:152)

128. **(B)** The pelvis is a bony basin formed by the two hipbones, the ossa coxae, and sacrum and coccyx of the vertebral column. It serves as a support of the vertebral column and for articulation with the lower limbs.
(34:124; 36:1248)

129. **(B)** The talus is the uppermost tarsal bone. It is the only bone of the foot that articulates with the tibia and fibula. It is surrounded on one side by the medial malleolus of the tibia and on the other side by the lateral malleolus of the fibula.
(38:171)

130. **(C)** Fracture of the femur usually occurs at the neck of the femur. It is inherently weakened by the angular junction with the shaft.
(34:126)

131. **(D)** The tibia is the larger medial bone of the lower leg. It bears the major portion of the weight on the leg. Another name is shinbone.
(38:171)

132. **(A)** The fibula is a long, slender, twisted bone on the lateral side of the tibia. It does not articulate with the femur. Its head articulates with the lateral aspect of the upper end of the tibia below the level of the knee joint.
(38:171)

133. **(B)** The head of the femur fits into a lateral depression in the os coxae (the acetabulum), forming a joint. It is held in place by a ligament and by tough fibrous capsule surrounding the joint.
(34:125)

134. **(A)** The patella, or kneecap, is a small, triangular bone anterior to the knee joint. It is a lens-shaped sesamoid bone situated in front of the knee in the tendon of the quadriceps femoris muscle.   *(38:171)*

135. **(B)** A muscle located at the front of the leg which acts on the foot is the tibialis anterior. It is responsible for dorsiflexion and inverts the foot.   *(38:260)*

136. **(B)** Fascia is a fibrous membrane covering, supporting and separating muscles. It unites the skin with the underlying tissue. It may be superficial or deep.   *(36:603)*

137. **(A)** Keratin is a tough protein substance in hair, nails, and horny tissue. It is insoluble in water, weak acids, or alkalies. It is unaffected by most proteolytic enzymes.   *(36:893)*

138. **(D)** The sebaceous glands are saclike or alveolar in structure. They are also called oil glands. They secrete sebum, a fatty secretion.   *(36:537)*

139. **(B)** There are two categories of membranes: epithelial and connective tissue. The epithelial is further divided into mucous membrane, which lines tubes and other spaces that open to the outside of the body, and serous membrane, which lines closed cavities within the body.   *(27:29–30)*

140. **(A)** The skin consists of two principal layers. The outer, thinner portion is called the epidermis. The epidermis is cemented to the inner, thicker connective tissue known as the dermis.   *(38:106)*

141. **(B)** The sweat glands secrete continuously, but so slowly that the droplets of moisture evaporate before they become visible. This type of sweating is called insensible perspiration.   *(34:84)*

142. **(A)** Long bones consist of a rodlike shaft with knoblike ends. The longest bone in the body is the femur. Another name is the thighbone.   *(38:171)*

143. **(D)** A condyle is a rounded protuberance found at the point of articulation with another bone. The distal end of the femur has large condyles. These condyles articulate with the tibia at the knee joint.   *(34:126)*

144. **(C)** Osteoporosis is a condition commonly seen in old age. It is characterized by a generalized loss of bone substance. Bone becomes brittle and the condition is very painful. Total hip replacement is a frequent procedure to improve mobility of patients with this disorder.   *(34:100)*

145. **(A)** The ends of long bones are called epiphyses. They have a somewhat bulbous shape which provides roomy areas for muscle attachments and gives stability to the joints.   *(34:95)*

146. **(C)** The dermis has a framework of connective tissue. It contains many blood vessels, nerve endings, and glands. It is known as the true skin.   *(38:106)*

147. **(B)** Osteoblasts are cells responsible for forming new bone during growth and repair. The root word *blast* means a germ or bud. It denotes an immature cell that later develops into a specialized form.   *(38:125)*

148. **(B)** The shaft of a long bone is called the diaphysis. It is a cylinder consisting mainly of compact bone. It is the main portion of the bone.   *(38:125)*

149. **(B)** The pigment granules called melanin give the skin its color. They are found in the epidermis. Melanin protects the body by screening out harmful ultraviolet sunrays.   *(38:65, 108)*

150. **(C)** The membrane that covers the bones is periosteum. It is adherent to the bone. It is a dense covering (white and fibrous) essential for bone growth, repair, and nutrition.   *(38:125)*

151. **(C)** Connective tissue is divided into three types: areolar, adipose, and reticular. Areolar tissue lies between organs and muscle, supporting blood vessels and nerves.   *(34:66)*

152. **(A)** Aponeurosis is a flat, fibrous sheet of connective tissue which serves to attach muscle to bone or other tissue at their point of origin or insertion. It may sometimes serve as fascia.   *(36:118)*

153. **(B)** Organs are called viscera. The membrane attached to the organs is the visceral layer. The visceral cavity contains the viscera.   *(36:1858)*

154. **(D)** The olfactory organs contain the smell receptors. They consist of various supporting cells in addition to the sensory receptors.   *(38:374)*

155. **(D)** The lens is a transparent, colorless structure in the eye which is biconvex in shape. It is enclosed in a capsule. It is capable of focusing rays so that they form a perfect image on the retina.   *(36:942)*

156. **(A)** The purpose of the iris is to regulate the amount of light entering the eye. The pupil is the contractile opening in the center of the eye.   *(38:382)*

157. **(D)** The iris is a thin, muscular diaphragm that is seen from the outside as the colored portion of the eye.   *(38:382)*

158. **(B)** The optic nerve carries visual impulses received by the rods and cones in the retina to the brain. This is the second cranial nerve.   *(38:333)*

159. **(B)** The eyeball has three separate coats or tunics. The outermost layer is called the sclera and is made of firm, tough connective tissue. It is known as the white of the eye.   *(38:379)*

160. **(C)** Aqueous humor is a watery, transparent fluid found in the anterior chamber and in the posterior chamber of the eye. It helps maintain the eye's conical shape and assists in focusing light rays. The posterior cavity lies between the lens and the retina and contains a jellylike substance called vitreous humor which helps prevent the eyeball from collapsing.   *(38:383)*

161. **(A)** The internal ear consists of the cochlea. This contains the sensory receptors for hearing. It also contains the vestibule and the semicircular canals which contain the receptors for equilibrium and sense of position.   *(36:510)*

162. **(B)** The eyeball is divided into three layers: fibrous tunic, vascular tunic, and the retina or nervous tunic. The fibrous (outer coat) is divided into two regions, posterior is the sclera and anterior is the cornea. The vascular (middle) layer is composed of the choroid which nourishes the retina, the ciliary body, and the iris. The nervous tunic (inner) is the retina.   *(38:379-382)*

163. **(A)** The projecting part of the ear is known as the pinna. It is also called the auricle. It is a trumpet-shaped flap of elastic cartilage covered by thick skin.   *(38:387)*

164. **(C)** Normally the air pressure on the two sides of the eardrum is equalized by means of the eustachian tube. This connects the middle ear cavity and the throat. This allows the eardrum to vibrate freely with the incoming sound waves.   *(38:389)*

165. **(D)** Near the exterior opening of the external ear, the canal contains a few hairs and specialized sebaceous glands called ceruminous glands. They secrete cerumen (ear wax).   *(38:387-388)*

166. **(B)** Conjunctiva is the mucous membrane that lines the eyelids and covers the anterior surface of the globe, except for the cornea. It is reflected onto the eyeball.   *(36:372)*

167. **(A)** The peripheral nervous system contains the 12 cranial and 31 spinal nerves and their branches to the entire body. This is outside of the central nervous system.   *(38:268)*

168. **(C)** The automatic nervous system is divided into the sympathetic nervous system and the parasympathetic nervous system.   *(38:268)*

169. **(D)** There are 31 pairs of spinal nerves. Each nerve is attached to the spinal cord by two roots, the dorsal root and the ventral root. By pairs there are 8 cervical, 12 thoracic, 5 lumbar, 5 sacral, and 1 coccygeal.   *(38:301)*

170. **(D)** The trigeminal nerve is the great sensory nerve of the face and head. It has three branches that carry general sense impulses. The third branch is joined by motor fibers to the muscles of chewing (mastication).   *(38:335)*

171. **(C)** The acoustic nerve, VIII, contains special sense fibers for hearing as well as balance from the semi-circular canal of the internal ear. It is also called the vestibulocochlear.   *(38:336)*

172. **(B)** The cerebellum is located immediately below the back part of the cerebral hemispheres. It is connected with the other parts of the brain by means of the bridgelike pons.   *(38:318)*

173. **(C)** It is in the cerebral cortex that all thought, association, judgment, and discrimination takes place. The voluntary movements are also controlled here.   *(27:86)*

174. **(A)** The cerebellum aids in coordinating the voluntary muscles, helps maintain balance in standing, walking, and sitting, and aids in maintaining muscle tone.   *(38:331)*

175. **(A)** Neurons are composed of a cell body containing the nucleus, with the addition of threadlike projections of the cytoplasm known as the nerve fibers. Neurons are the functional units of the nervous system which conduct impulses from one part of the body to another.   *(27:86; 38:269)*

176. **(B)** The parietal lobe contains the sensory area in which the general senses such as pain, touch, and temperature are interpreted.   *(27:87)*

177. **(D)** The lobes of the cerebral hemispheres are named after the skull bones that they underlie. They are the frontal, parietal, temporal, and occipital lobes.   *(21:347)*

178. **(D)** Within the medulla are three vital reflex centers of the reticular system. The cardiac center regulates heart beat, the respiratory center adjusts the rate and depth of breathing, the vasoconstrictor center regulates the diameter of the blood vessels.   *(38:318)*

179. **(B)** The largest part of the brain is the cerebrum, which is divided into the two cerebral hemispheres (a right and a left side). It is supported on the brainstem.   *(38:324)*

180. **(B)** The meninges are three layers of connective tissue that surround the brain and the spinal cord to form a complete enclosure. The outermost layer of these membranes is called the dura mater. The second layer around the brain and spinal cord is the arachnoid membrane. The third layer is the pia mater.
(38:310; 27:96)

181. **(A)** Between the arachnoid and the pia mater is the subarachnoid space. This is where the cerebral fluid circulates. *(38:290)*

182. **(B)** Within the brain are four fluid-filled spaces called the ventricles. They are cavities that communicate with each other, with the central canal of the spinal cord, and with the subarachnoid space. *(38:310)*

183. **(B)** At the end of the auditory canal is the tympanic membrane. It is also known as the eardrum. This membrane serves as the lateral wall of the tympanic cavity. *(36:1792)*

184. **(D)** The cochlea looks like a small shell. It is a tube coiled for about two and a half turns into a spiral, around a central axis of the bone. *(34:325)*

185. **(D)** At the end of the auditory canal is the tympanic membrane, or eardrum. It serves as a boundary between the external auditory canal, or meatus, and the middle ear cavity. It is thin and semitransparent. *(38:389)*

186. **(D)** The left ventricle is a heavy, thick-walled pump which pumps blood out into the largest blood vessel in the body, the aorta. The entrance of the aorta is guarded by the aortic semilunar arch. *(34:365)*

187. **(B)** The main function of hemoglobin is that it is the iron-containing pigment of red blood cells. Its function is to carry oxygen from the lungs to the tissues. The average in adult males is 14 to 18 and in adult females 12 to 16. *(36:746)*

188. **(B)** Plasma is the straw-colored liquid portion of the blood in which the various solids are suspended. *(36:1313)*

189. **(D)** The hematocrit is the volume percentage of red blood cells in whole blood. The average in adult males is 47% and in adult females 42%. *(36:730)*

190. **(B)** White blood corpuscles, leukocytes, act as scavengers. By doing so, they help combat infection. They are phagocytic (ingest particulate substances). *(36:947)*

191. **(A)** The hand receives blood that courses through the subclavian artery. This becomes the axillary artery in the armpit. *(27:149–150)*

192. **(C)** The differential white count (an estimate of the percentage of each type of white cell) is done using a stained blood slide. Some blood diseases and inflammatory conditions can be recognized this way.
(36:212)

193. **(A)** Incompatibility of blood transfusions may be due to either the plasma or red cells of the donor's blood. The red cells of the donor's blood may become clumped or held together in bunches. This process is called agglutination. *(36:48)*

194. **(C)** Platelets are particles that bring about the process of clotting. Platelets are also known as thrombocytes. Platelets number 200,000 to 300,000. *(36:1316)*

195. **(A)** Erythrocytes are mature red blood cells. Their function is to carry oxygen and carbon dioxide but also aid in acid-base balance of the blood and in the formation of bile pigments. *(36:571)*

196. **(D)** Hemolysis is the destruction of red blood cells with liberation of hemoglobin. *(34:354–355)*

197. **(B)** The erythrocytes are formed in the red bone marrow. This is the connective tissue found inside the numerous small spaces of the spongy parts of all bones. They are mature red cells which have the primary function of carrying oxygen and carbon dioxide. *(27:124)*

198. **(C)** A normal adult has an average of 5,000 to 10,000 leukocytes per cubic millimeter of circulating blood, or about 1 leukocyte to 700 erythrocytes. A high white blood count is indicative of infection. *(36:948)*

199. **(B)** The saphenous vein is the longest vein in the body. The greater saphenous vein, which is superficial, extends up the medial side of the leg, the knee, and the thigh. At the groin it empties into the femoral vein. *(38:508)*

200. **(C)** In the bend of the elbow, the median cubital vein ascends from the cephalic vein on the lateral side of the arm to the basilic vein on the medial side. It is the preferred vein for venipuncture. *(38:504)*

201. **(A)** The external iliac artery changes to the femoral in the thigh. This vessel branches off in the thigh and then becomes the popliteal artery at the back of the knee joint. It subdivides below the knee. The popliteal vein is also behind the knee. *(38:508)*

202. **(B)** The superior mesenteric artery, which is the largest branch of the abdominal aorta, carries blood to most of the small intestine as well as to the first half of the large intestine. The much smaller inferior mesenteric artery, which is located near the end of the abdominal aorta, supplies the major part of the large intestine and the rectum. *(38:498)*

203. **(A)** The azygos vein drains the veins of the thorax and empties into the superior vena cava just before the latter empties into the heart. It also may serve as bypass for the inferior vena cava that drains blood from the lower body. *(38:506)*

204. **(D)** The palmar arch forms the union of the radial and ulnar arteries in the hand. It sends branches to the hand and the fingers, via the distal arteries. *(38:496)*

205. **(D)** Blood from the face, scalp, and superficial regions of the neck is drained by the internal and external jugular vein. The internal jugulars flow into the superior vena cava. The external jugulars flow into the subclavian veins. *(38:504)*

206. **(C)** Blood is supplied to the heart by the right and left coronary arteries. Branches of these two arteries encircle the heart and supply all the parts of the myocardium. Branches lead to the atrial and ventricular myocardium. *(38:496)*

207. **(B)** Impulses that start at the sinoatrial node spread through the atrial muscle fibers, producing atrial contractions. When the impulses reach the A-V node they are relayed to the ventricles via the bundle of His and the Purkinje fibers, producing synchronized contraction of the ventricles. *(38:463-465)*

208. **(A)** The right primary bronchus is more vertical, shorter, and wider than the left. As a result, foreign objects in the air passageways are more likely to enter it than the left and frequently lodge in it. *(38:550)*

209. **(D)** The spleen is an organ containing lymphoid tissue designed to filter blood. It is frequently damaged in abdominal trauma causing it to rupture. This causes severe hemorrhage which requires prompt splenectomy. *(38:525)*

210. **(B)** Most parts of the body receive branches from more than one artery. The junction of two or more vessels supplying the same body region is an anastomosis. Anastomosis between arteries provides alternate routes for the blood. If a vessel becomes occluded, circulation is taken over by the alternate route; this is known as collateral circulation. *(38:482)*

211. **(D)** The arch of the aorta sends off three large branches: the brachiocephalic, the left common carotid, and the left subclavian artery. The coronaries arise from the ascending aorta. *(38:496)*

212. **(B)** The left and right carotid arteries supply the head and neck. The external carotid supplies the right side of the thyroid, tongue, throat, face, ear, scalp, and the dura mater. *(38:496)*

213. **(A)** Pericardium forms the outermost layer of the heart wall. It also lines the pericardial sac. It is a loose fitting membrane. Pericarditis is an inflammation of the lining. *(38:457)*

214. **(C)** The posterior cerebral arteries help to form an arterial circle at the base of the brain called the circle of Willis, which creates a connection between the vertebral artery and internal carotid artery systems. It equalizes blood pressure to the brain and provides alternate routes for blood to the brain. *(38:496)*

215. **(B)** The external iliac arteries continue into the thigh, where the name of these tubes is changed to femoral. Both femorals go to the genitals and abdominal wall. Other branches run to the thigh and become the popliteal (back of the knee). *(38:500)*

216. **(D)** The descending aorta travels through the thorax, branching off to supply the thoracic organs and structure. It then passes through the diaphragm into the abdomen, supplying the abdominal organs via numerous branches. It terminates at the level of the fourth vertebra, dividing into the two common iliac arteries, which supply the pelvis and lower extremities. *(38:498-500)*

217. **(D)** Arteries and veins can be subdivided into two groups. The pulmonary vessels, including pulmonary artery and pulmonary veins, eliminate carbon dioxide from the blood and replenish its supply of oxygen. *(38:458)*

218. **(C)** The right ventricle pumps the venous blood dropped into it from the right atrium and sends it to the lungs, via the pulmonary veins. *(36:1844)*

219. **(A)** The right atrium is a thin-walled space that receives the venous blood returning from the body tissues. This blood is carried in the veins, which are the blood vessels leading to the heart. *(36:52; 27:138)*

220. **(A)** The contractions of the heart are synchronized and their rate is controlled by specially modified muscular tissue. The sinoatrial node, the pacemaker, is found in the right atrial wall near the opening of the superior vena cava. *(38:463)*

221. **(D)** The arterioles lead into a vast network of very fine blood vessels, the capillaries. These are the blood vessels that permeate the tissues and service the body cells directly. They play a key role in regulating blood flow from arteries to capillaries. *(38:483-484)*

222. **(D)** The human heart is a double pump. The two sides are completely separated from each other by a partition called the septum. *(38:457)*

223. **(B)** The left atrioventricular is called the bicuspid valve. This valve also has a third alternate name, the mitral valve. *(36:194)*

224. **(D)** The tricuspid valve (right atrioventricular) closes at the time the right ventricle begins pumping in order to prevent blood from going back into the right atrium. It has three flaps or cusps and is between the right atrium and the right ventricle. *(38:459–461)*

225. **(B)** The endocardium, which lines the inner surface of the heart cavity, is a thin, delicate membrane composed of endothelial cells. It covers the valves, surrounds the chordae tendineae, and is continuous with the lining membrane of the large blood vessels. *(38:457)*

226. **(A)** The spleen is located in the upper left hypochondriac region of the abdomen and is normally protected by the rib cage. It is between the fundus of the stomach and the diaphragm. *(38:524)*

227. **(C)** The thymus plays a key role in the formation of antibodies in the first few weeks of life and in the development of immunity. It also stimulates the formation of lymphocytes. Its role in immunity is to help produce cells that destroy invading microbes and manufactures antibodies. *(38:425–426)*

228. **(C)** Cervical nodes, located in the neck, often become enlarged during upper respiratory infections as well as certain chronic disorders. They act as filters keeping bacteria out of the blood stream. *(27:105)*

229. **(A)** Lymph, lymph vessels, lymph nodes, tonsils, thymus, and the spleen make up the lymphatic system. Its function is to drain from the tissue-spaces protein containing fluid that escapes from the blood capillaries. It also transports fats from digestive tract to the blood. *(38:520)*

230. **(D)** The s-shaped bend where the colon crosses the brim of the pelvis and enters the pelvic cavity (where it becomes the rectum) is the sigmoid colon. It begins at the left iliac crest, projects toward the midline and terminates at the rectum. *(38:618)*

231. **(A)** The large intestine has little or no digestive function. It serves to reabsorb water and electrolytes. It also forms and stores feces until defecation occurs. *(38:619–621)*

232. **(D)** The narrow, distal part of the large intestine is called the anal canal. The rectum is the last 8 inches of the gastrointestinal tract. The terminal 2 inches is the anal canal. *(38:618)*

233. **(A)** The large intestine is approximately 5 feet long and 2.5 inches in diameter. It extends from the ileum to the anus. It is divided into the cecum, colon, rectum, and anal canal. *(38:618)*

234. **(C)** The omentum is a double fold of peritoneum attached to the stomach and connecting it to certain abdominal viscera. The portion that is suspended from the greater curvature of the stomach and covers the intestines like an apron is the greater omentum. It contains fat, aids in keeping the intestines warm, and aids in localizing infection. *(36:1159)*

235. **(B)** The beginning (proximal) portion of the large intestine is the cecum. It hangs below the ileocecal valve. It is a blind pouch 2.5 inches long. *(38:618)*

236. **(C)** To the cecum is attached a small blind tube known as the appendix. It is a twisted, coiled tube, 3 inches in length. *(38:618)*

237. **(A)** The gallbladder stores bile between meals and releases it when stimulated by gastric juice, fatty foods, and the hormone cholecystokinin. Bile is produced in the liver. The gallbladder stores and concentrates bile. *(38:610)*

238. **(B)** When the gallbladder contracts, it ejects concentrated bile into the duodenum. Bile is forced into the common bile duct when it is needed. *(38:610)*

239. **(B)** Pancreatic juice leaves the pancreas through the pancreatic duct, the duct of Wirsung. The pancreatic duct unites with the common bile duct from the liver and gallbladder and enters the duodenum in a small raised area called the ampulla of Vater. *(38:604–606; 36:1840)*

240. **(D)** The peritoneum is a serous membrane which covers the surface of most of the abdominal organs and lines the abdominal wall. Parietal peritoneum lines abdominal and pelvic walls. The visceral invests the abdominal organs. *(36:1269)*

241. **(B)** The hepatic duct joins the slender cystic duct from the gallbladder to form the common bile duct. The common bile duct and the pancreatic duct enter the duodenum in a common duct, hepatopancreatic. *(38:606)*

242. **(A)** The folds in the lining of the stomach are called rugae. They disappear as the stomach fills with food. *(38:598)*

243. **(D)** The bile pigments, bilirubin and biliverdin, are products of red blood cell breakdown and are normally excreted in bile. If their excretion is prevented, they accumulate in the blood and tissues, causing a yellowish tinge to the skin and other tissues. This condition is called obstructive jaundice. *(38:609)*

244. **(A)** The pancreas is an oblong, fish-shaped gland which consists of a head, tail, and body. The head rests in the curve of the duodenum, and its tail touches the spleen. It is linked to the small intestine by a series of ducts.   *(38:604)*

245. **(D)** The ileum, the last section of the small intestine, joins with the large intestine and the ileocecal valve. It is about 2 feet long.   *(38:610)*

246. **(B)** The ileocecal sphincter or valve joins the large intestine to the small intestine.   *(38:612)*

247. **(C)** The duodenum receives secretions from the pancreas and the liver. The duodenum originates at the pyloric sphincter and extends 10 inches where it merges with the jejunum.   *(21:498, 504–507; 38:610)*

248. **(B)** Parasympathetic impulses stimulate certain stomach cells to release a hormone called gastrin. This causes the gastric glands to increase their secretory activity.   *(38:602)*

249. **(A)** Gastric juice has two main components, hydrochloric acid and enzymes such as pepsin.   *(36:665)*

250. **(A)** The cardiac region of the stomach is a small area near the esophageal opening. The rounded portion is the fundus. The central portion, the body, and the narrow inferior region is the pylorus.   *(38:597)*

251. **(D)** The mesentary is a double-layered peritoneal structure shaped like a fan. It connects to the posterior abdominal wall. The long edge is attached to the small intestine. Between the two layers of membrane are blood vessels, nerves, and other structures which supply the intestine.   *(27:191)*

252. **(B)** The balloonlike portion of the stomach that extends above the level of the junction with the esophagus is called the fundus. Above the fundus is the cardia. Below is the body.   *(38:597)*

253. **(D)** At the end of the pyloric canal, the muscular wall is thickened, forming a circular muscle called the pyloric sphincter. Pyloric stenosis is a narrowing of the pyloric sphincter which prevents food from passing through.   *(38:597)*

254. **(C)** The pharynx is divided into three parts: the nasopharynx, the oropharynx, and the laryngopharynx. Another name is the throat. It is funnel-shaped and is 5 inches long.   *(38:543)*

255. **(A)** Exocrine glands secrete their products into ducts (tubes) that empty at the surface of the covering or lining or directly on a free surface. The secretions of these glands are mucus, perspiration, oil, wax, and digestive enzymes.   *(38:84)*

256. **(D)** The esophagus is a straight, collapsible tube about 10 inches long. It lies behind the trachea. It pierces the diaphragm at the esophageal hiatus.   *(38:594)*

257. **(A)** The esophagus penetrates the diaphragm through an opening, the esophageal hiatus, which then empties into the stomach.   *(38:594)*

258. **(C)** The posterior region, or root, of the tongue is anchored to the hyoid bone. It is covered with lymphatic tissue called the lingual tonsils. Its functions are mastication, speech production, and taste.   *(36:1745)*

259. **(D)** The soft palate forms an arch that extends posteriorly and downward as a cone-shaped projection. This is called the uvula. It is composed of connective tissue, muscle, and mucous membrane.   *(36:1824)*

260. **(A)** Masses of lymphatic tissue, called the pharyngeal tonsils, are located on the posterior wall of the pharynx above the border of the soft palate. When hypertrophied, it is called adenoid.   *(36:1281)*

261. **(B)** Infected tonsils can become so swollen that they block the passageways of the pharynx, thus interfering with breathing and swallowing. There is also danger of infection spreading from the throat to the middle ear because the eustachian tube and the middle ear are continuous.   *(21:485)*

262. **(C)** The incisors are chisel-shaped; their sharp edges serve to bite off large pieces of food. They are referred to as either being central or lateral.   *(38:592)*

263. **(D)** The cuspids (canines) are cone-shaped with pointed tips. They grasp and tear at food. Cuspids have only one root.   *(38:592–593)*

264. **(A)** The molars, or bicuspids, have a flattened surface and are used for grinding and crushing food. Upper molars have three roots. Lower molars have two roots.   *(38:593)*

265. **(B)** The alveolus portion of the tooth refers to the tooth socket or canal. It is a small hollow or cavity.   *(36:64)*

266. **(A)** The parotid glands are the largest of the salivary glands. They are located just under and in front of each ear. Each secretes into the oral cavity via the parotid duct.   *(38:591)*

267. **(B)** The sublingual glands are located under the tongue. They open into the floor of the mouth in the oral cavity.   *(38:591)*

268. **(A)** The liver is the largest gland in the body. It is divided into left and right segments or lobes. It is located unter the diaphragm. Bile is one of its chief products.   *(38:606)*

269. **(D)** The glomerulus is a cluster of capillaries located on one end of the nephron. It is a rounded mass of nerves or blood vessels.   *(38:786)*

270. **(D)** The ureter expands to form a collecting basin for urine in the renal pelvis. Tubelike extensions project from the renal pelvis into active kidney tissue to increase the area for collection. These are calyces.   *(38:661)*

271. **(A)** The kidneys have three functions: excretion, water balance, and regulation of acid-base balance. The bladder is a reservoir for urine.   *(38:658)*

272. **(C)** Contractions of the muscular coat of the ureters produce peristaltic waves, which transport urine along the ureters. Peristalsis is the main function of the musculature.   *(38:677)*

273. **(C)** The smooth, triangular area at the bottom of the bladder is the trigone. The two ureters enter the bladder at the upper corners of the trigone. Urine flows out of the urethra through the internal orifice located at the bottom of the trigone.   *(38:678)*

274. **(B)** The male urethra is about 20 cm long and is divided into three sections. It serves as both excretory and reproduction functions, carrying either semen or urine.   *(34:562)*

275. **(B)** The kidneys are positioned retroperitoneally. This means that they are behind the parietal peritoneum and against the deep back muscles. Other retroperitoneal structures are the ureters and the suprarenal glands.   *(38:657)*

276. **(B)** The functional unit of the kidney is the nephron.   *(38:661)*

277. **(C)** Blood is supplied to the kidney through the renal artery, which arises from the abdominal aorta. The renal arteries transport about one-fourth of the total cardiac output to the kidney.   *(38:665)*

278. **(A)** The medulla is the inner part of the kidney. Within the medulla are the renal pyramids. The outer layer is the cortex.   *(38:658)*

279. **(A)** The hilus is a concave indentation of the medial surface of the kidney through which all structures that enter or leave the kidney pass. These structures are the renal artery, the renal vein, and the renal pelvis.   *(38:658)*

280. **(D)** The cortex is the outer part or layer of the kidney. The inner layer is the medulla.   *(38:658)*

281. **(C)** The male urethra passes through the prostate gland (prostatic portion), the pelvic floor (membranous portion), and along the length of the penis (cavernous portion).   *(38:705)*

282. **(A)** Normal constituents of urine are sodium, urea, ammonia, uric acid, and creatinine. Abnormal constituents are glucose, ketone bodies, albumin, pus, bile, and pigments or calculi.   *(34:555–556)*

283. **(B)** Uremia is the toxic condition of the blood, caused by a buildup of urea and other toxins. It is the result of a disturbed kidney function as seen in nephritis.   *(36:1807)*

284. **(D)** Retention is a failure to void urine and may be due to an obstruction, a nervous contraction of the urethra, or a lack of sensation to void.   *(38:678)*

285. **(C)** Lack of control over micturition or urination is termed incontinence. This may be the result of tumor growths or herniation of adjacent structures pressing on the bladder.   *(38:676)*

286. **(A)** Urine empties from the bladder through a tube called the urethra. It emerges at an opening on the exterior surface of the body called the urinary meatus.   *(34:562)*

287. **(D)** The bladder is a temporary reservoir for urine. It is a hollow muscular organ situated in the pelvic wall cavity posterior to the symphysis pubis.   *(38:677)*

288. **(A)** If an ovum is fertilized by a sperm cell, it most often occurs in the upper third of the uterine tubes. Fertilization may occur at any time up to 24 hours following ovulation. The ovum, whether fertilized or not, descends into the uterus within several days.   *(34:638)*

289. **(D)** In the female, the area located between the vagina and the anus is the perineum. It is cut during delivery (episiotomy) to prevent rectal tearing and subsequent damage.   *(38:720)*

290. **(A)** Within the labia majora lie the labia minora. They border the vestibule. They are thin, highly vascular, and contain sebaceous glands but no hair or sweat glands.   *(38:719)*

291. **(B)** The small protuberance that contains specialized nerve endings sensitive to stimulation is the clitoris. It lies about 1 inch superior to the urethral orifice and is homologus to the male penis.   *(34:627)*

292. (D) The uterus has three layers. The outer layer is the peritoneal covering, which is continuous with the peritoneum of the broad ligament. The middle layer is thick and muscular and is called the myometrium. The inner layer is vascular mucous membrane called endometrium. *(34:743-744)*

293. (A) The vestibule of the vulvae is the space that is enclosed by the labia minora. The vagina opens into the posterior portion and the urethra opens in the midline, anterior to the vagina and behind the clitoris. *(38:720)*

294. (C) Anatomic divisions of the uterus are: the dome-shaped portion above the uterine tubes, called the fundus; the major tapering central portion, called the body; and the inferior narrowed portion projecting into the vagina, called the cervix. *(38:713)*

295. (B) There is no direct connection between the ovaries and the fallopian tubes. The ova are swept into the tubes by a current in the peritoneal fluid, produced by small, fringelike projections from the abdominal openings of the tubes. These are known as fimbriae. *(38:709)*

296. (B) Ovulation, stimulated by the hormones of the anterior pituitary gland, causes the mature follicle to swell and rupture. When this occurs the follicular fluid and egg cells ooze from the surface of the ovary and enter the peritoneal cavity. They are then propelled to the nearby uterine tube, through which they enter the uterus. *(38:711-713)*

297. (C) A pair of greater vestibular glands, the Bartholin's glands, are found on each side of the vaginal orifice. They secrete a mucous substance that moistens and lubricates the vestibule and vagina. *(34:624)*

298. (C) The ovaries are attached to the broad ligament of the uterus by a fold or peritoneum called the meso-varian, anchored to the uterus by the ovarian ligaments, and attached to the pelvic wall by the suspensory ligament. *(38:709)*

299. (D) The spermatic cord is the supporting structure of the male reproductive system. It consists of veins, arteries, lymphatics, nerves, the vas deferens, and a small band of skeletal muscle called the cremaster muscle. *(38:704)*

300. (B) A loose fold of skin called the prepuce, or foreskin, begins just behind the glans penis and extends forward as a sheath. In the female, it is formed where the labia minora unite and cover the entire body of the clitoris. *(38:707, 719)*

301. (A) The distal end of the penis is slightly enlarged and is called the glans, meaning shaped like an acorn. Covering the glans is the foreskin. *(38:707)*

302. (D) The vas deferens unites with the duct of a seminal vesicle outside the prostate gland. The fusion of these two ducts forms an ejaculatory duct, which passes through the prostate gland and empties into the urethra through a slitlike opening. *(38:704-705)*

303. (B) The prostate gland surrounds the posterior urethra just below the urinary bladder. In older males it often enlarges, causing interference with the excretion of urine. It is doughnut-shaped and about the size of a chestnut. *(38:706)*

304. (A) The secretion of the seminal vesicles adds bulk to the semen and helps nourish and protect the delicate sperm. *(34:618)*

305. (D) The vas deferens, the seminal duct, is a muscular tube that begins at the lower end of the epididymis and passes upward at the medial side of the testes to become part of the spermatic cord. It passes through the inguinal canal, enters the abdominal cavity, and ends behind the bladder where it joins (outside the prostate) with the seminal vesicle, forming the ejaculatory duct. *(38:704-706)*

306. (B) Sperm mature in the epididymis, where they are stored and propelled toward the urethra during ejaculation. *(38:703)*

C. MICROBIOLOGY

307. (C) Leeuwenhoek had an untiring interest in the microscopic world. This was a simple microscope consisting of one lens, similar to a magnifying glass. *(2:70; 37:58)*

308. (D) Lister speculated that if Pasteur was right about the presence of microorganisms in the air, such organisms could also enter surgical wounds and cause sepsis and wound deterioration. He used carbolic acid (phenol) to kill bacteria. *(37:8)*

309. (C) The smallest of this group, the viruses, are mere particles when compared in size to molecules and are structurally simpler than any microorganisms. Viruses are parasites of other biologic groups. *(37:14)*

310. (D) Weakened pathogens are genetically changed by attenuation so that they are no longer pathogenetic. Attenuation means a weakened, less pathogenic organism. *(39:18)*

311. **(A)** A spore is a reproductive cell. They possess a thick wall enabling the cell to withstand unfavorable environmental conditions. The spores of bacteria are difficult to destroy because of their resistance to heat and require prolonged exposure to high temperatures to destroy them.   *(36:1610)*

312. **(C)** Osmosis allows the passage of the solvent–usually water–to pass through the membrane from the region of lower concentration of solute to the region of higher concentration. This tends to equalize the concentration of the two solutions.   *(36:1182)*

313. **(D)** The majority of microbes are aerobes. This means they grow and flourish in the presence of oxygen.   *(8:61)*

314. **(D)** Leukocytes known as phagocytes rush to a wound to engulf and destroy the bacteria present. Phagocytosis means "cell eating."   *(8:153)*

315. **(D)** Most of the contagious airborne diseases are due to respiratory pathogens carried in the droplets of moisture to susceptible individuals. Colds, influenza, and mumps are contagious diseases. Streptococci are nonmotile.   *(8:134)*

316. **(B)** Artificially acquired active immunity occurs when a person receives a vaccination (vaccine). This causes specific antibodies to be produced. The person then forms antibodies against the pathogen before exposure to the disease.   *(8:162)*

317. **(C)** *Staphylococcus aureus* is commonly present on skin and mucous membranes, especially those of the nose and the mouth. It is gram positive. They are the cause of suppurative conditions such as boils, carbuncles, and internal abscesses.   *(36:1617–1618)*

318. **(A)** Members of the *Clostridium* group of bacteria are anaerobes (live and grow in absence of oxygen). *C. perfringens* is responsible for gas gangrene which causes death of soft tissue due to loss of blood supply. Substances released from dying and dead cells produce nutrients for bacteria.   *(37:515; 36:78)*

319. **(A)** Antigens are the body's third line of defense. The immune response produces antibodies in response to the presence of particular substances known as antigens.   *(8:149)*

320. **(B)** Microorganisms can multiply in the blood. Infection of bacterial origin carried through the bloodstream is referred to as bacteremia or septicemia. Microorganisms invade from a focus of infection in the tissue.   *(2:74)*

321. **(B)** Autogenous vaccines are pathogens that are killed, then injected into the same person to induce production of antibodies.   *(8:163)*

322. **(A)** When the exudate of the inflammatory process is thick and yellow with a large number of leukocytes, it is called purulent or suppurative. Suppurative is to form or generate pus.   *(36:1658; 39:155)*

323. **(C)** Parasitism causes some damage to the host. Depending on the parasite and the circumstances, the damage may be slight or fatal. A parasite lives in, upon, or at the expense of another organism.   *(8:83)*

324. **(A)** Binary fission is the splitting of each cell into two new daughter cells, each of which contains the same components as the original parent cell. It is an asexual reproduction. Each develops into a complete individual.   *(36:622)*

325. **(B)** The production of toxic products by pathogens is the most influential factor in their pathogenicity. Pathogenicity is the ability of an organism to cause disease.   *(8:118)*

326. **(C)** The organisms and vectors are usually species specific. Mosquitoes carry yellow fever, ticks transmit Rocky Mountain spotted fever, and flies transfer typhoid bacillus.   *(13:13)*

327. **(B)** This increase may account for the relatively high virulence of pathogens in a hospital environment, where the population is continually changing.   *(8:110)*

328. **(B)** The unbroken skin acts as a mechanical barrier to pathogens. Only when it is cut, scratched, or burnt can pathogens gain entrance. Mucous membranes entrap invaders.   *(8:151)*

329. **(D)** All personnel directly or indirectly involved in surgery are responsible for the control of the environment and equipment.   *(8:124)*

330. **(B)** The easiest access route for infectious organisms is the respiratory tract. It is also the most difficult route to control. Skin and hair of the patient and OR team are also contributory.   *(2:79)*

331. **(C)** Spirilla are short little forms of bacteria, with one to three fixed curves in their rigid bodies. Those with only one curve resemble a comma. Their bodies are fairly rigid, shaped as a cork screw.   *(37:77)*

332. **(C)** Operative technique is one of the most important factors influencing wound healing. Meticulous technique should be used. It is advisable to isolate wound closure materials so that every wound (infected or not) may be closed with previously unused, sterile instruments.   *(2:85)*

333. **(A)** Rubella (German measles) is caused by the rubella virus. It is a serious disease because it is related to serious birth defects and maternal infection during the first trimester of pregnancy. The results could be a stillborn birth, or deafness, cataracts, heart defects, or mental retardation.   *(37:499)*

334. **(B)** The system in common use today was developed by a Swedish botanist named Carl Von Linne and is called the Linnaean system. It has been greatly modified and enlarged but remains the basis for modern classification or microorganisms.   *(37:12)*

335. **(D)** Bacteria are unicellular and the simplest form of cell organization. Protozoa are the most complex although still unicellular. Fungi molds are multicellular and complex.   *(37:12–14)*

336. **(A)** Herpes simplex, commonly called "cold sores," is an example of a viral agent capable of latent periods where the virus is not multiplied. It remains intact until stress encourages growth. Also known as fever blisters. Appearance associated with trauma, sun, hormonal changes, and emotional upset.   *(37:499)*

337. **(C)** Local irritation causes the small blood vessels to dilate and become more permeable. The tissue spaces become engorged with fluid and edema results. In inflammation there is pain, redness, heat, swelling, vasodilation, and disturbance of function.   *(8:156)*

338. **(C)** *Clostridium tetani* is the causative organism of tetany or lockjaw. Commonly found in soil contaminated with animal fecal waste. Protection is provided by receiving tetanus toxoid to stimulate antibodies against tetanus toxins. A booster may be given when a dangerous wound is received.   *(36:343; 37:516–517)*

339. **(C)** Many bacteria possess flagella, which are threadlike appendages that provide the cell with the capacity for motion. Some species of bacteria with many flagella produce wavelike motions across culture medium.   *(37:79–80)*

340. **(A)** The specimen is first dyed with a solution of gentian violet and then fixed with an iodine solution. Bacteria retaining the purple color of the gentian violet are gram positive. Those that lose the first color are gram negative.   *(37:67–68)*

341. **(B)** Three basic shapes identify bacteria. Cocci (or singular, coccus) and spherical. Bacilli (singular, bacillus) are rodlike, and spirilla (singular, spirillum) are spiral-shaped.   *(37:12)*

342. **(B)** When the organisms of gas gangrene are introduced into tissues where conditions permit anaerobic multiplication, they utilize amino acids and carbohydrates freed from dead or dying cells.   *(37:515–516)*

343. **(C)** In nature, rickettsiae occur chiefly in insects such as lice, ticks, or mites. The disease is transmitted to its progeny and then transmitted to man by the insect bite. It is responsible for typhus, Rocky Mountain spotted fever, and Q fever.   *(37:271)*

344. **(A)** *Clostridium tetani* is found in soil contaminated with fecal animal waste. Improperly cleaned deep puncture wounds provides the anaerobic condition necessary for its growth. DPT immunization (which includes tetanus toxoid) is a standard immunization. A booster of toxoid may be given when a dangerous wound is received.   *(37:516–517)*

345. **(B)** Koch developed many of the technical methods of cultivation, staining, and animal experimentation vital to the study of microorganisms and the interpretation of their behavior as agents of disease.   *(37:351)*

346. **(B)** A beta hemolytic streptococci, *Streptococcus pyogenes,* sometimes leads to the development of rheumatic fever. This disease usually is expressed as an arthritis. It frequently also takes the form of an inflammation of the heart, causing damage to the valves.   *(37:556)*

347. **(C)** Anaphylactic shock is the state of collapse resulting from injection of a substance to which one has been sensitized. It is a severe allergic reaction. Death may occur if emergency treatment is not given.   *(8:173)*

348. **(A)** The milk or colostrum secreted for a few days following delivery contains maternal antibodies, which also protect the infant in early months of life. This is natural, acquired, passive, immunity.   *(8:163–164)*

349. **(D)** *Staphylococcus aureus* is associated with skin infections such as boils, carbuncles, furuncles, and impetigo.   *(37:267)*

350. **(B)** *Pseudomonas aeruginosa* most frequently found in burns, presents very difficult problems because the organism is generally resistant to many clinically useful antibiotics.   *(37:515)*

351. **(B)** Scarlet fever is caused by the streptococci. The toxin causes a pink-red skin and high fever. The tongue is spotted with strawberrylike appearance. Complications like deafness can occur.   *(37:580)*

352. **(A)** Endogenous substances are produced or arise within a cell or organism. The antonym of endogeny is exogeny – outside an organism. It concerns spore formation within the bacterial cell.   *(37:545)*

353. **(B)** A carrier is an infected person, circulating free in the community, who has few or no symptoms, and communicates the infection in transit. Diseases such as diphtheria, salmonellosis, epidemic pneumonia, and streptococcal infections may be spread. *(37:352)*

354. **(C)** The number of cases in a community increases and decreases at times, but the disease never dies out completely and thus is considered endemic. Incidence depends on a balance of factors including environment, humidity, the group's naturally acquired immunity, and the virulence of the pathogen. *(8:114)*

355. **(A)** A member of the defense team is the protective protein interferon. It is secreted by tissue cells, when they are infected by viruses. *(8:140)*

356. **(D)** Joseph Lister, an English surgeon, saw great value in Pasteur's work. He searched for a chemical to combat surgical infections, and utilizing a phenolic solution developed his "Principles of Antiseptic Surgery." *(2:71)*

357. **(D)** Although *Escherichia coli* is a universal member of the normal intestinal flora, it has been associated with gastroenteritis in infants. More recently it has been identified as the culprit responsible for "Montezuma's revenge," "Delhi belly," and other gastrointestinal disturbances. *(37:264)*

358. **(A)** *Staphylococcus aureus* produces furuncles, carbuncles, and impetigo. One of the most important skin invaders, it produces tissue destruction and abscesses if it escapes localization. *(37:492)*

359. **(B)** A wound with a poor blood supply (ischemia) can lead to necrosis (death of tissue). The death of soft tissue due to loss of blood supply is gangrene. Gas gangrene caused by *Clostridium perfringens* develops with ischemia and necrosis. *(37:515)*

360. **(D)** The autoimmune response in which the body produces disordered immunologic responses against itself, causing tissue injury. Certain forms of glomerular nephritis, rheumatoid arthritis, myasthenia gravis, and scleroderma are considered autoimmune diseases. *(8:174)*

361. **(D)** Gas gangrene is caused by the microorganism *Clostridium perfringens*. *(37:515)*

362. **(D)** Fibrolysin, an enzyme produced by hemolytic streptococcus may dissolve fibrin and delay localization of a streptococcal infection. The body attempts to wall off an abscess by means of a membrane that produces surrounding induration (hardened tissue) and heat. *(2:75)*

363. **(D)** Mucus-to-mucus contact is often called the venereal route because gonorrhea and syphilis are transmitted only this way. However, many other pathogens use this route. *(8:133)*

364. **(A)** The most resistant form of microbial life is the endospore. Spores have a thick wall making them difficult to destroy. This enables them to withstand unfavorable conditions such as heat. They require a prolonged exposure time to high temperatures to destroy them. *(37:515; 36:1610)*

D. PHARMACOLOGY

365. **(D)** Levophed is a potent peripheral vasoconstrictor. It is useful in peripheral vascular collapse, such as hypotension or cardiogenic shock. Some of its actions are similar to epinephrine. *(2:208)*

366. **(A)** Demerol (meperidine HCl) is an analgesic for moderate pain to severe pain. It produces analgesia and sedation. It may produce temporary euphoria. *(17:97)*

367. **(A)** A Seng-Staken Blakemore tube is used to control esophageal hemorrhage. Pressure is exerted on the cardiac portion of the stomach and against bleeding esophageal varices by a double balloon tamponade. It is a three element gastric tube. *(36:1783)*

368. **(D)** Oxycel's hemostatic action is caused by the formation of an artificial clot by cellulose action as it reacts with blood. It increases in size to form a gel and stops bleeding. It is used dry. *(2:245)*

369. **(C)** Protamine sulfate is a proteinlike substance which by itself is an anticoagulant. When given in the presence of heparin, each neutralizes the anticoagulant activity of the other. Thus it is a heparin antagonist. *(36:1393)*

370. **(C)** Vitamin K in its natural form or in its synthetic form (menadione) is essential in the synthesis of prothrombin by the liver. It is especially useful in conditions in which prolonged bleeding time is the result of a low concentration of prothrombin in the blood. It has an antihemorrhagic factor. *(36:1862)*

371. **(B)** Of the following inhalation anesthetic agents, penthrane is nonexplosive and nonflammable; diethyl ether is flammable; cyclopropane is highly explosive; sodium pentothal is an intravenous barbiturate used for anesthesia induction. *(2:171)*

372. **(C)** Pitocin is used to induce active labor or to increase the force or rate of existing contractions during delivery. It may be given postpartum to prevent or control hemorrhage. It acts on the uterus. *(17:95)*

373. **(B)** Ergotamine is useful in the treatment of migraine headaches because of its vasoconstricting effects on cerebral vessels. It also stimulates uterine contractions.
(36:568)

374. **(A)** Alpha chymotrypsin (alfachymar) is an enzyme which dissolves the zonules holding the lens in place. It is injected behind the iris into the posterior chamber to dissolve the filaments that hold the lens.
(17:435)

375. **(A)** Pilocarpine is a miotic. A miotic causes the pupil to contract.
(17:435)

376. **(B)** Tetracaine provides rapid, brief, and superficial anesthesia. It is widely used as a local ocular anesthetic. It is the generic name for Pontocaine.
(17:435)

377. **(B)** Hyaluronidase is commonly added to an anesthetic solution. This enzyme increases diffusion of the anesthetic through the tissue, thereby improving the effectiveness of the block.
(32:663)

378. **(C)** Renografin and hypaque sodium are contrast media used for radiography of the biliary tract, kidney, and other internal structures. When injected, shows as white on x-ray.
(17:97)

379. **(C)** Traumatic injuries to the eye are treated with antibiotics for infection and steroids for inflammation. Celestan and Decasone are two anti-inflammatory eye drugs.
(17:435)

380. **(B)** Ventricular fibrillation requires prompt defibrillation and CPR. It is rapidly fatal, since respiratory and cardiac arrest follow quickly unless successful defibrillation is effected.
(2:201–202)

381. **(C)** Propranolol hydrochloride (Inderal) is useful in ventricular fibrillations or tachycardia. It is hazardous when cardiac function is depressed. It is also used in treating hypertension.
(36:1389)

382. **(A)** Calcium chloride is useful in profound cardiovascular collapse. It increases myocardial contractility, enhances ventricular excitability, and prolongs systole. Calcium cannot be given together with sodium bicarbonate because a precipitate forms from the mixture.
(2:208)

383. **(A)** Dextran is used to expand plasma volume in emergency situations resulting from shock or hemorrhage. It acts by drawing fluid from the tissues. It remains in the circulatory system for several hours. (2:144)

384. **(D)** Avitene is a microfibrillar collagen hemostatic agent. It is an adjunct to hemostasis when conventional methods are ineffective. It is an absorbable topical agent of purified bovine collagen and it must be applied in its dry state. It is very expensive.
(17:95)

385. **(D)** Sodium bicarbonate counteracts metabolic acidosis generated during time without oxygen. It elevates the pH of the blood. It restores the bicarbonate ion.
(2:208)

386. **(B)** An ounce (fluid, apothecaries) is a measure for liquids. It is equal to 29.6 milliliters thus 30 ml.
(36:1192)

387. **(A)** During the induction phase, the patient retains an exaggerated sense of hearing until the last moment. Thus it is essential that all personnel in the room remain as quiet as possible. (17:65)

388. **(A)** Allergic reaction effects can be reduced by antihistamines, epinephrine, or corticosteroids. Antihistamines oppose the action of histamine. (36:61, 105)

389. **(A)** Keflin is an antibiotic. It blocks cell wall synthesis. It is used in treatment of respiratory, genitourinary, skin, soft tissue, bone and blood infections caused by many organisms both gram positive and gram negative.
(17:96)

390. **(D)** Balanced salt solution is an eye irrigant. It is used to keep the eye moist during surgery. It is supplied in a sterile solution. (17:435)

391. **(B)** Pontocaine is tetracaine hydrochloride. It is commonly used for infiltration and nerve block.
(2:184)

392. **(D)** One gram is equivalent to 15 grains. It equals approximately the weight of a cubic centimeter or a milliliter of water. (36:701)

393. **(A)** Pitocin is used to produce firm contractions and decrease uterine bleeding. It induces parturition (afterbirth). (36:1200)

394. **(D)** Heparin may be used locally or systemically to prevent thrombosis during vascular operative procedures. When a vessel is completely occluded during surgery, heparin is often injected directly. Heparinized saline irrigation may also be used. The dosage and concentration may vary according to the surgeon's preference. The saline used *must* be injectable saline.
(32:426)

395. **(C)** Sedatives are drugs that soothe and relieve anxiety. The only difference between a hypnotic and a sedative is one of degree. A hypnotic produces sleep while a sedative provides mild relaxation. It is quieting and tranquilizing. (36:1540)

396. **(C)** The drug which reverses the effect of muscle relaxants is neostigmine. It is also known as Prostigmin. *(32:137; 36:1392)*

397. **(C)** The basic unit of weight in the apothecaries' system is the grain, which originally meant a grain of wheat. The abbreviation is gr. *(36:701)*

398. **(B)** Antipyretics are the drugs used to reduce body temperature and thereby reduce the possibility of tissue damage. It is an agent that reduces fever. *(36:108)*

399. **(C)** Steroids reduce tissue inflammation and postoperative swelling. Examples are Decadron, Cortisporin ophthalmic ointment. In eye surgery they are applied topically to reduce post-op swelling. In plastic surgery, in and around the site in patients who tend to form keloids. *(17:100)*

400. **(A)** Anectine is an ultra-short acting muscle relaxant of rapid onset used mostly in intubation. It can be used for continuing relaxation in a dilute solution. Also known as succinylcholine chloride. *(2:176)*

401. **(B)** Excess carbon dioxide from the patient's breath is absorbed by soda lime in a container on the machine. Soda lime is a chemical absorber. This is used in a closed anesthesia system. *(2:169)*

402. **(D)** Spinal anesthesia is an extensive nerve block, sometimes called a subarachnoid block. It affects the lower spinal cord and nerve roots. It is used for lower abdominal or pelvic procedures. *(2:180–181)*

403. **(A)** Naloxone (Narcan) is a drug that prevents or reverses the action of morphine and other opiates. This is a specific narcotic antagonist. *(36:1096)*

404. **(D)** Tetracaine produces surface anesthesia in eye surgery and is available in an 0.5% concentration for this use. Pontocaine is the tradename for this topical solution. *(17:435)*

405. **(B)** Neuroleptanalgesia describes the state resulting from the combination of a narcotic (potent analgesic) and a tranquilizer (neuroleptic). When the narcotic tranquilizer combination is reinforced by use of an anesthetic such as nitrous oxide, the state is referred to as neuroleptanesthesia. This is a state of balanced anesthesia. *(2:167)*

406. **(B)** Rapid induction is an advantage of nitrous oxide induction. It gives poor relaxation, possible excitement or laryngospasm. Good in procedures requiring little relaxation. *(2:170)*

407. **(C)** Extubation is precarious for the patient who may cough, jerk, or experience a spasm of the larynx from tracheal stimulation. Hypoxia is a common complication. It is a deficiency in oxygen. *(2:169–170)*

408. **(C)** Serial monitoring of blood gases is indispensable in evaluating pulmonary gas exchange and acid-base balance. Either or both arterial or venous blood gas determination can be monitored. It is a chemical analysis of the blood for concentrations of oxygen and carbon dioxide. *(2:188)*

409. **(D)** Methylprednisolone (Medrol) is an adrenal corticosteroid drug. Corticosteroids prevent the normal inflammatory response thus it is anti-inflammatory. In eye surgery, they reduce the resistance to the eye to invasion by bacterial viruses and fungi. *(36:1043; 32:661)*

410. **(C)** A minim equals 1/60 of a fluidram or 0.06 milliliter. One cc equals approximately 30 minims. *(36:1055–1056)*

411. **(B)** Lidocaine (xylocaine) is used intravenously for treatment of cardiac arrhythmias particularly ventricular in nature. It is used before, during, and after cardiac procedures, in cardiac arrest, and in treatment and prevention of irritability in myocardial infarct. *(17:98; 2:183–184)*

412. **(B)** Nitrous oxide (laughing gas) would probably be considered an ideal anesthetic if it were more potent. It is nonexplosive, safe, and pleasant smelling. It has a rapid induction and recovery. *(2:170)*

413. **(B)** Local anesthesia depresses superficial nerves and blocks the conduction of pain impulses from a specific area or region. The sensory nerves are the first affected. *(2:178)*

414. **(B)** Adrenalin is another name for epinephrine. *(17:98)*

415. **(C)** Less anesthesia is needed in induced hypothermia, when the body temperature has been lowered below normal limits. It reduces metabolic rate and oxygen needs of tissues. Bleeding is decreased and less anesthesia is used. *(2:191)*

416. **(C)** Cocaine is unrivaled in its power to penetrate mucous membrane to produce surface anesthesia. Onset is immediate. It also causes vasoconstriction to reduce bleeding. Administration is only topical because of its high toxicity. *(2:183)*

417. **(D)** Pentothal (thiopental sodium) is potent; it has a cumulative effect and very rapid uptake from the blood. It is the most frequently used. It is short acting. *(2:172)*

418. **(A)** One fluid ounce is equal to 29.573 ml. One milliliter is equal to 1 cubic centimeter. Thus 30 cc is equal to 1 ounce.   *(36:1055, 1905)*

419. **(D)** The drug Marcaine has a duration of 2 to 3 times longer than lidocaine or Carbocaine and provides prolonged pain relief. It has high potency of long duration. It affords prolonged pain relief following block.
(2:184)

420. **(D)** Induction with cyclopropane is both pleasant and rapid. It is a very potent gas that is seldom used. It is highly explosive.   *(2:170)*

421. **(B)** One ounce equals 29.6 ml. There are 16 ounces in 1 pint or approximately 473.2 ml. Thus the closest answer is 500 ml.   *(36:1192, 1303)*

422. **(C)** The closed method of anesthesia allows complete rebreathing of expired gases. This system provides for maximal conservation of heat and moisture, increases resistance to breathing and reduces cost and confines gas to machine.   *(2:169)*

423. **(B)** This is the excitement stage. It varies greatly with individuals but begins with loss of consciousness. In this stage there is sometimes irregular breathing and limb movements.   *(32:132)*

424. **(A)** Morphine sulfate relieves moderate to severe pain. It is an analgesic. It produces mood elevation, euphoria, and relief of fear and apprehension as well.
(17:97)

425. **(C)** Both atropine and scopolamine are given for parasympathetic depressant action, mainly for the inhibition of mucus secretion. The patient complains of dry mouth after their administration however they should not be given any water to drink if they are NPO.
(2:165)

426. **(D)** Naloxone (Narcan) is a specific narcotic antagonist. It has no depressant action.   *(2:165)*

427. **(D)** Balanced anesthesia is a technique whereby the properties of anesthesia (hypnosis, analgesia, and muscle relaxation) are produced in varying degrees by a combination of agents.   *(2:167)*

428. **(A)** An epidural is used for anorectal, vaginal, perineal, and obstetrical procedures. Injection is made into the space surrounding the dura mater within the spinal canal (the epidural space).   *(2:182)*

429. **(C)** Miochol is a myotic (mytocic, miotic) used to constrict the pupil. It reduces intraocular pressure or in cataract surgery helps prevent the loss of the vitreous.
(17:435)

430. **(B)** Epinephrine is added to a local anesthetic when a highly vascular area is to be injected. It causes vasoconstriction at the operative site. This holds the anesthetic in the tissue, prolongs its effect, and minimizes local bleeding.   *(17:63)*

E. WOUND HEALING

431. **(A)** Abdominal sepsis may result from enteric flora if the intestine is perforated or transected. Among the genera included as enterics is *E. coli.*   *(2:76; 17:263)*

432. **(C)** Although Halsted is well known for his fine-pointed hemostat, use of the penrose drain, and rubber gloves, he is best known for his "Principles of Tissue Handling." The silk suture technique which he developed, although modified, is still in use today.   *(2:238)*

433. **(C)** Third degree burn includes the skin with all its epithelial structures and subcutaneous tissue destruction. It is characterized by a dry, pearly white, or charred-appearing surface void of sensation. The destroyed skin forms a parchmentlike eschar over the burned area.   *(2:453)*

434. **(D)** Vitamin K is an aid to the clotting of blood in vessels. It reduces the possibility of hemorrhage during surgery. It is given to patients who have been on anticoagulant therapy.   *(2:244)*

435. **(C)** Surgical incisions are in the classification of incised wounds. Incised means to cut as with a sharp instrument.
(36:832)

436. **(C)** The inflammatory response is the body's attempt to neutralize and destroy toxic agents at the site of injury and prevent their spread. After injury the metabolic rate increases, quickening heartbeat. More blood circulates to area causing dilation of vessels. Large amount of blood in the area is responsible for redness.
(17:99)

437. **(B)** After debris and infected or contaminated tissue is removed by debridement, the wound is irrigated thoroughly. Devitalized tissue is removed because it acts as a culture medium. The third intention of healing requires debridement.   *(2:242)*

438. **(D)** Serum or blood clots can form in this dead space and prevent healing by keeping the cut edges of the tissue separated. It is the space caused by separation of wound edges that have not been closely approximated.
(2:239)

439. **(A)** Closure that is too tight or under tension causes ischemia, a decrease in blood supply to the tissues, and eventually tissue necrosis.   *(2:242)*

440. **(B)** When the collagen in the tissue remains constant, the fiber pattern reforms cross-links to increase tensile strength in the tissue. Tensile strength is the ability of the tissues to resist rupture.   *(2:239)*

441. **(C)** Retention sutures or stay sutures give support to wounds prone to dehiscence until healing. They may be used as a precautionary measure to prevent wound disruption.   *(2:263)*

442. **(A)** In operations on the blood vessels or heart, and in patients who have a history of thromboembolic disease, anticoagulants are used. The dosage is adjusted to minimize the tendency of blood to clot in vessels, yet not to lead to excessive bleeding during or following the operation.   *(2:243)*

443. **(B)** Proud flesh is wound healing by "second intention," where fibrous bands form after the healing is complete. It is an overgrowth of granulation tissue.   *(32:127)*

444. **(B)** Collagen is a protein substance that is secreted from fibroblasts to form fibers of connective tissue. It is found in connective tissue and represents about 30% of total body protein.   *(2:239; 36:352)*

445. **(A)** Fibrinogen unites with thrombin (a product of prothrombin and thromboplastin) to form fibrin, which is the basic structural material of blood clots. It is essential for the clotting of blood.   *(2:243)*

446. **(B)** A cicatrix or scar is formed by the intertwining of cells surrounding the capillaries and binding together in final closure of a wound. It is a scar left by a healing wound.   *(36:331)*

447. **(B)** Hypoxia is deficiency of oxygen. It is a decreased concentration in the inspired. Hypoxemia is insufficient oxygenation of the blood.   *(36:814)*

448. **(B)** Vitamin C aids in connective tissue production and strong scar formation.   *(32:126)*

449. **(C)** A keloid is a scar formation of the skin following trauma or surgical incision. The result is a raised, firm, thickened red scar. Blacks are especially prone to keloids.   *(36:897)*

450. **(B)** Wound healing is basically collagen synthesis; therefore, any agent such as a steroid that interferes with cellular metabolism has a deleterious effect on healing.   *(2:240)*

451. **(B)** Healing by granulation (second intention) involves a wound that is either infected or one in which there is excessive loss of tissue. The skin edges cannot be adequately approximated. Generally, there is suppuration (pus formation), and abscess, or necrosis.   *(32:125)*

452. **(C)** Tetanus is an acute infectious disease caused by *Clostridium tetani,* which grows anaerobically at the site of an injury. All contaminated traumatic injuries must be treated for tetanus bacillus.   *(2:242)*

453. **(C)** Healing by third intention implies that suturing is delayed for the purpose of walling off an area of gross infection involving much tissue removal as in debridement of a burn when suturing is done later. Third intention of healing means that two opposing granulation surfaces are brought together. Granulation usually forms a wide, fibrous scar.

          (32:125–126)

454. **(D)** Loose sutures prevent the wound edges from meeting and create dead spaces, which discourage healing. Tight sutures or closure under tension causes ischemia.   *(2:242)*

455. **(C)** Second-intention healing is commonly referred to as granulation healing. This form of wound healing takes longer than first intention, but is equally as strong once healed. It heals from the inside to the outside surface.   *(32:125)*

F. GROSS ANATOMY

The Eye

456. cornea
457. anterior chamber
458. posterior chamber
459. pupil
460. lens
461. iris
462. vitreous humor
463. retina
464. choroid
465. sclera
466. optic nerve

The Ear

467. auricle
468. auditory canal
469. tympanic membrane
470. malleus
471. incus
472. stapes
473. cochlea
474. semicircular canal
475. auditory nerve

The Heart

476. left auricle
477. left ventricle
478. right ventricle

479. right auricle
480. superior vena cava
481. inferior vena cava
482. arch of aorta
483. ascending aorta
484. right coronary artery
485. left coronary artery

The Respiratory System

486. nasal cavities
487. nasopharynx
488. oropharynx
489. laryngopharynx
490. epiglottis
491. larynx
492. trachea
493. bronchi
494. lung
495. bronchioles
496. pleura
497. diaphragm

The Urinary System

498. adrenal glands
499. kidney
500. ureters
501. urinary bladder
502. urethra

The Kidney

503. fibrous capsule
504. medulla
505. cortex
506. pyramid

507. papilla
508. calyx
509. renal pelvis
510. ureter

The Brain

511. cerebrum
512. cerebellum
513. thalamus
514. hypothalamus
515. pituitary gland
516. pons
517. medulla oblongata

The Skull

518. parietal bone
519. occipital bone
520. temporal bone
521. sphenoid bone
522. mandible
523. maxilla
524. zygomatic bone
525. lacrimal bone
526. nasal bone
527. frontal bone

Forms of Bacteria

528. coccus
529. diplococcus
530. streptococcus
531. staphylococcus
532. bacillus
533. spirillum
534. spirochete

CHAPTER 2

Patient Care
Questions

Directions: Each of the questions or incomplete statements below is followed by four suggested answers or completions. Select the best answer in each case.

A. PRE-OP ROUTINE

1. The preoperative urinalysis test done on Mrs. McSweeney indicates that the specific gravity is 1.050. This

A. is within normal range
B. is below normal range and she is dehydrated
C. is above normal range and she is dehydrated
D. is indicative of sugar in the urine

2. A type and cross-match is done

A. on all surgical patients
B. if the surgeon anticipates in advance of the operation that blood loss replacement may be necessary
C. on all hospital patients
D. in the OR

3. Lynne D. is scheduled for surgery. Her hematocrit reading is 40% of whole blood volume. This is

A. within normal range
B. below normal range
C. above normal range
D. inconclusive

4. Cross-matching of blood refers to

A. blood typing
B. blood grouping
C. blood compatibility
D. Rh factor determination

5. Gary Robert is on anticoagulant drugs. Which of the following tests may be done to check the clotting time of his blood?

A. serum amylase
B. complete blood count
C. bleeding time
D. prothrombin time

6. Preoperative chest x-rays

A. are not necessary for the surgical patient
B. are necessary only for the thoracic surgical patient
C. are necessary only on the surgical patient with a chronic cough
D. should be done on all surgical patients

7. An electrocardiogram is

A. an electrical recording of heart activity
B. an x-ray defining heart structures
C. an x-ray of the cardiac portion of the stomach
D. a stress test on the heart

8. After being scheduled in the OR for a routine tonsillectomy, the nurse checking the chart of Kim A. notes that the hemoglobin is 9.0 g. This reading is

A. within normal range
B. below normal range
C. above normal range
D. inconclusive

9. A microscopic blood exam that estimates the percentages of each type of white cell is called a

A. red blood count
B. white blood count
C. differential blood count
D. blood grouping

10. Protein or albumin in the urine indicates

A. urinary tract infection
B. diabetes
C. acute or chronic renal disease
D. dehydration

11. A bacteria count of 10,000/ml of urine is

A. within normal range
B. below normal range
C. above normal range
D. of no significance

12. The normal pH of urine is

A. 6
B. 12
C. 18
D. 24

13. The sequential multiple analyzer (SMA) test is done to determine

A. blood typing
B. an evaluation of electrolytes, enzymes, blood urea nitrogen, blood sugar, cholesterol, and triglyceride in the blood
C. percentages of each type of white blood cell in the blood
D. total red and white blood counts

14. Which procedure is *not* absolutely necessary in patient identification?

A. identification by the anesthesiologist, who checks the wristband, chart, and operating schedule
B. identification by the surgeon before administration of an anesthetic
C. identification by the circulating nurse, who checks the wristband, chart, and operating schedule
D. identification by the scrub nurse before the procedure begins

15. In the event that a child needs emergency surgery and the parents cannot be located to sign the permission

A. no permission is necessary
B. permission is signed by a court of law
C. permission is signed by the physician
D. a written consultation by two physicians other than the surgeon will suffice

16. Informed consent means that the patient

A. has been informed about what will be done and gives his or her permission
B. is of age and mentally capable of signing
C. signs voluntarily after the procedure, complications, and postoperative course are explained
D. is protected from unauthorized surgery

17. Kristin Lee is scheduled for an appendectomy. After completing this procedure the surgeon decides to remove a mole from her shoulder while she is still under anesthesia. No permission was obtained for this. The circulating nurse should

A. report it to the anesthesiologist
B. report it to the chief of surgery
C. report it to the supervisor or proper administrative authority
D. let the surgeon proceed since it is his responsibility to obtain the consent

18. The surgical consent form can be witnessed by each of the following *except*

A. the surgeon
B. a nurse
C. an authorized hospital employee
D. the patient's spouse

19. Scott A. is premedicated and is brought to the operating room for a cystoscopy and an open reduction of the wrist. Upon arrival in the operating room, it is observed that he has only signed for the cystoscopy. The correct procedure would be to

A. cancel surgery until a valid permission can be obtained
B. have him sign for the additional procedure in the operating room
C. ask him verbally for his consent and have witnesses attest to it
D. let the surgeon make the decision as to whether surgery could be done

20. A general consent form is

A. a form authorizing all treatments or procedures
B. a form for all patients having general anesthesia
C. a form for all patients having hazardous therapy
D. another name for an operative permit

21. The ultimate responsibility for obtaining consent lies with the

A. operating room supervisor
B. circulating nurse
C. surgeon
D. unit charge nurse

22. Upon arrival in the operating room, a patient tells the nurse that she knows she will die during the procedure. The nurse should

A. reassure the patient that this will not happen
B. tell the patient that everyone feels that way
C. record it on the operative record
D. report it to the surgeon

23. If a patient requests to see a clergyman upon his or her arrival in the OR

A. the clergyman should be sent for
B. reassure patient that he or she can see him when he or she wakes up
C. make a note on the chart for the floor nurse to contact him
D. tell the patient he or she has nothing to fear

24. Which statement concerning the obese surgical patient is false?

A. obesity may delay the healing process because of poor vascularity
B. obese patients have an increased incidence of postoperative wound infection
C. adipose tissue retains anesthetic drugs longer
D. obese patients are more prone to hyperglycemia

25. The patient has received preoperative medication. The action to be taken when this patient complains of dry mouth, thirst, and requests water would be

A. provide the patient with unlimited water for thorough hydration
B. restrict water to 2 ounces
C. restrict fluids completely and explain reason for action of medication
D. report to the surgeon immediately

26. A myelogram is an x-ray of the

A. muscle wall of uterus
B. spinal canal
C. meninges
D. pupils of the eye

27. When is the surgical consent signed?

A. before induction
B. in the holding area
C. the morning of surgery
D. before administration of pre-op medications

28. The normal pH of blood is

A. 3.5–4.5
B. 7.35–7.45
C. 14.25–16
D. 25.5–31.25

29. A bowel prep for intestinal surgery is

A. mechanical and chemical
B. mechanical
C. chemical
D. eliminated

B. TRANSPORTATION

30. When using a patient roller, how many people are necessary to move the patient safely and efficiently?

A. two
B. three
C. four
D. five

31. During transportation of a patient in traction to the OR

A. the weights are removed and left in the patient's room
B. the weights are removed and placed on the stretcher shelf
C. the weights are not removed but supported so as not to swing
D. the weights are not removed but are carried by the transporter

32. When moving the patient from the OR table, who is responsible for guarding the head and neck from injury?

A. circulating nurse
B. scrub nurse
C. anesthesiologist
D. surgical technician

33. To move the patient from the transport stretcher to the OR table,

A. one person stands at the head, one at the foot, while the patient moves over
B. one person stands next to the stretcher, one adjacent to the OR table, while the patient moves over
C. one person stands next to the stretcher, stabilizing it against the OR table, while the patient moves over
D. one person may stand next to the OR table and guide the patient toward him, if stretcher wheels are locked

34. Stretchers used for transport should be equipped with

A. siderails and restraining strap
B. siderails, restraining strap, and brakes
C. siderails, restraining strap, brakes, and pillow
D. siderails, restraining strap, brakes, and IV pole

35. When moving a patient with a fracture in the OR, all of the following are true except

A. extra personnel are necessary
B. support of the extremity should always be from below the site of fracture
C. lifters on the affected side support the fracture
D. the surgeon should be present

36. Personnel transporting the patient to the OR should

A. talk to the patient to prevent nervousness
B. treat the patient gently and not appear to be in a hurry
C. transport the patient as quickly as possible to prevent patient anxiety
D. transport the patient as quickly as possible so there is no delay in the schedule

37. Occult blood means it is

A. from the upper GI tract
B. from the lower GI tract
C. microscopic
D. grossly evident

38. All of the following patients may be transported to the OR in their beds *except* the

A. ICU patient
B. orthopedic fracture patient
C. comatose patient
D. elderly patient

39. In order to avoid compromising the venous circulation, the restraint or safety strap should be placed

A. at knee level
B. at the midthigh area
C. 2 inches above the knee
D. 2 inches below the knee

40. Herbert A., a patient with a fractured femur, is being moved to the OR table. Who is responsible for supporting and protecting the fracture site?

A. the nurse assistant
B. the physician
C. the circulating nurse
D. the scrub nurse

C. POSITIONING

41. Crossing the patient's arms across his or her chest may cause

A. pressure on the ulnar nerve
B. interference with circulation
C. postoperative discomfort
D. interference with respiration

42. The desirable position for better visualization in the lower abdomen or pelvis is

A. Fowler's
B. reverse Trendelenburg
C. Trendelenburg
D. Kraske

43. A precaution always taken when the patient is in supine position is to

A. place the pillows under the knees for support
B. place the safety strap 3 to 4 inches below the knee
C. place the head in a headrest
D. protect the heels from pressure on the OR table

44. The femoral nerve could be injured if

A. the patient in lithotomy position is not padded properly
B. retractors are used carelessly during pelvic surgery
C. the safety strap is placed on too tightly
D. the Mayo stand leans on the patient's feet

45. Untying the patient's gown assures

A. easier access to the operative site
B. easier access for the IV administration
C. no pressure on any nerves
D. no interference with respiration

46. In order to prevent strain to the lumbosacral muscles and ligaments when the patient is in lithotomy position,

A. the buttocks must not extend beyond the table edge
B. the legs must be placed symmetrically
C. the legs must be at equal height
D. a pillow should be placed under the sacral area

47. The anesthesia screen is placed on the OR table

A. after induction and positioning
B. after induction and before positioning
C. after the patient is placed on the OR table
D. anytime before draping

48. The lithotomy position requires each of the following *except*

A. patient's buttocks rest along the break between the body and leg sections of the table
B. stirrups are at equal height on both sides of the table
C. stirrups are at the appropriate height for the length of the patient's legs to maintain symmetry
D. each leg is raised slowly and gently as it is grasped by the toes

49. Which position would be the most desirable for a pilonidal cystectomy or a hemorrhoidectomy?

A. lithotomy
B. Kraske
C. knee-chest
D. modified prone

50. A position often used in cranial procedures is called

A. Fowler's
B. Kraske
C. Trendelenburg
D. lithotomy

51. Another name for the Kraske position is

A. prone on an adjustable arch
B. lateral
C. knee-chest
D. jackknife

52. The purpose of the kidney elevator is to

A. increase the space between the lower ribs and iliac crest
B. increase the space between the ribs
C. stabilize the patient
D. support the body in the flexed position

53. Which of the following is *not* a requirement when the patient is in prone position?

A. the safety belt is placed above the knees
B. the arms may be on armboards, alongside the body, or raised above the head
C. the head is turned to the side
D. bolsters are placed under the axillae and alongside the chest

54. In positioning for laminectomy, rolls or bolsters are placed

A. horizontally, one under the chest and one under the thighs
B. longitudinally to support the chest from axilla to hip
C. longitudinally to support the chest from sternum to hip
D. below the knees

55. Why is the table straightened before closing a kidney incision?

A. to facilitate easier respirations
B. to create better approximation of tissues
C. to facilitate better circulation
D. to prevent nerve damage

56. All of the following are requirements of the Kraske position *except*

A. patient is prone with hips over the break of the table
B. a pillow is placed under lower legs and ankles
C. a padded knee strap is applied 2 inches above knees
D. arms are tucked in at sides

57. The patient is never positioned until the

A. surgeon gives his permission
B. anesthesiologist gives his permission
C. scrub nurse is in the room
D. circulating nurse has finished all her preparatory duties

58. The placement of the patient in the operative position is the responsibility of the

A. surgeon
B. circulating nurse
C. circulating nurse, anesthesiologist, and surgeon
D. circulating nurse and surgeon

59. When using an armboard the most important measure is to

A. support the arm at the intravenous site
B. strap the patient's hand to it securely
C. avoid hyperextension of the arm
D. avoid hypoextension of the arm

60. Anesthetized patients should be moved slowly to

A. prevent fractures
B. prevent circulatory overload
C. allow the respiratory system to adjust
D. allow the circulatory system to adjust

61. If the patient is in supine position the circulator must always

A. place a pillow between the knees
B. place a pillow under the knees
C. see that the ankles and legs are not crossed
D. see that the thoracic area is padded adequately

62. Extreme positions of the head and arm can cause injury to the

A. cervical plexus
B. radial nerve
C. ulnar nerve
D. brachial plexus

63. Ulnar nerve damage could result from

A. poor placement of legs in stirrups
B. hyperextension of the arm
C. using mattress pads of varying thickness
D. placing an arm on an unpadded table edge

64. Which position would be used for a patient in hypovolemic shock?

A. modified Trendelenburg
B. reverse Trendelenburg
C. supine
D. dorsal recumbent

65. In prone position, the thorax must be elevated from the OR table to prevent

A. compromised respiration
B. pressure areas
C. circulatory impairment
D. brachial nerve damage

66. The anesthesiologist closes the eyelids of a general anesthetic patient for all of the following reasons *except* to

A. prevent drying of the eye
B. prevent the patient from seeing the procedure
C. prevent eye trauma
D. protect the eye from anesthetic agents

D. RELATED NURSING PROCEDURES

67. The initial count requires

A. a count of both plain and radiopaque sponges
B. that counts be done in the right-hand corner on the back table
C. that the count be done aloud by circulator and scrub
D. the scrub to count each item and report to the circulator for recording

68. If cardiac arrest occurs in the OR who is responsible for handling artificial ventilation?

A. the anesthesiologist
B. the circulating nurse
C. the surgeon
D. the scrub nurse

69. Sudden shortness of breath in a postoperative patient may be indicative of

A. pulmonary embolism
B. pleural effusion
C. emphysema
D. asthma

70. If a sponge pack contains an incorrect number of sponges, the circulating nurse should

A. take the pack out of the room immediately
B. document it on the count record
C. use if after adding or subtracting the correct number
D. return it to the original outer package and set it aside

71. In an instrument count

A. all instruments and parts must be counted
B. precounted sets eliminate the need for precase count
C. large bulky instruments need not be counted
D. count only instruments that will be used

72. Which is *not* an indication for use of suprapubic bladder drainage?

A. kidney operation
B. vaginal hysterectomy
C. prostatic surgery
D. urethral injuries

73. All of the following are helpful in keeping accurate account of sponges *except*

A. keep sponges separate from linen and instruments
B. keep needles separate from sponges
C. keep all sponges and tapes in a basin or close together on the field
D. keep a mental count of the number of sponges on the field at any given time

74. Amputated extremities are

A. sent to the pathology lab as are other specimens
B. preserved in formaldehyde
C. wrapped and refrigerated
D. placed in a dry container

75. Which pulse is checked during a cardiac arrest effort?

A. radial
B. carotid
C. pedial
D. rachial

76. Diastolic blood pressure refers to

A. the force created by the contraction of the left ventricle of the heart
B. the relaxation phase between heartbeats
C. the first sound heard when taking the pressure on a manometer
D. the high point of the cycle

77. Systolic blood pressure represents

A. the pressure in the heart chambers, great vein, or close to the heart
B. the relaxation phase between heartbeats
C. the low point of the cycle
D. the greatest force caused by contraction of the left ventricle of the heart

78. Subnormal temperature is known as

A. hyposalemia
B. hypotonia
C. hypovolemia
D. hypothermia

79. Airways should be

A. removed before the patient leaves the OR site
B. left in until the patient is fully awake and ready to return to his room
C. left in place until the patient breathes normally
D. removed only by the anesthesiologist

80. An anesthetic complication characterized by progressive elevation of body temperature is known as

A. malignant hypothermia
B. malignant hypervolemia
C. malignant hypersalemia
D. malignant hyperthermia

81. A drug used in the management of ventricular cardiac arrhythmias is

A. sodium bicarbonate
B. epinephrine
C. lidocaine
D. Levophed

82. Tachycardia is a/an

A. heartbeat over 100 beats per minute
B. irregular heartbeat
C. thready, weak heartbeat
D. heartbeat less than 60 beats per minute

83. The pulse of an athlete is generally

A. higher than that of the nonathlete
B. the same as that of the nonathlete
C. lower than that of the nonathlete
D. lowered following exercise

84. A pulse deficit refers to the difference between

A. the pulse before exercise and after exercise
B. the apical pulse rate and the peripheral pulse rate
C. the pulse rate before inspiration and after expiration
D. the radial pulse rate and the femoral pulse rate

85. The true configuration of the pulse is most accurately obtained at the

A. dorsalis pedis artery
B. femoral artery
C. radial artery
D. carotid artery

86. When observing the respiratory rate,

A. count each inspiration and expiration as one breath for 1 full minute
B. count each inspiration as one and each expiration as one for 1 full minute
C. count each rise of the chest and abdomen for at least 30 seconds
D. count each fall of chest and abdomen for 2 full minutes

87. A telethermometer monitors the body temperature during surgery. It can be placed in all of the following areas *except* the

A. rectum
B. esophagus
C. axilla
D. tympanic area

88. Dark blood in the operative field may indicate that the patient is

A. hyperkalemic
B. hypovolemic
C. hypotensive
D. hypoxic

89. The first and most important step for successful resuscitation in cardiac arrest is

A. the precordial thump
B. artificial ventilation
C. immediate opening of the airway
D. external cardiac compression

90. The responsibility of the scrub nurse in CPR is to

A. bring in the emergency cart
B. keep a record of all medication given
C. help with the intravenous and monitoring lines
D. give attention to the sterile field and the surgeon's needs

91. Morphine sulfate is used in advanced life support as a/an

A. treatment for acute pulmonary edema
B. vasoconstrictor
C. agent to counteract acidosis
D. diuretic

92. A drug used to treat severe bradycardia in the presence of hypotension is

A. Lasix
B. calcium chloride
C. lidocaine
D. atropine sulfate

93. A safety precaution used when a patient is being shocked with the defibrillator is

A. no one is to touch the patient or anything metallic in contact with the patient
B. available personnel gently but firmly support the extremities to protect the patient from injury
C. the person holding the electrodes does not touch the patient but anyone else can
D. the person holding the electrodes is the only one who may touch the patient

94. External cardiac compression

A. restores and maintains oxygenation
B. provides pulmonary ventilation
C. provides oxygen to vital tissues
D. provides peripheral pulse

95. When handling a syringe of medication to the surgeon for a local anesthetic, the scrub nurse should

A. ask the circulating nurse what solution he or she has
B. ask the circulator to show the vial to the surgeon
C. show the surgeon the vial that it came from
D. state the kind and percentage of the solution

96. When a local anesthetic is being used in the OR,

A. a registered nurse must check the label
B. the scrub person assumes full responsibility once the anesthetic is on the sterile field
C. the registered nurse dispenses it directly to the surgeon
D. the surgeon checks the label when it is poured

97. When cardiac arrest occurs, resuscitative measures must begin within

A. 2 minutes
B. 3–5 minutes
C. 2–7 minutes
D. 5–8 minutes

98. Who is responsible for recording all medications given during CPR in the OR?

A. the scrub nurse
B. the circulating nurse
C. the anesthesiologist
D. the surgeon's assistant

99. The body temperature taken orally is 98.6°F. What is it in Celsius?

A. 37°C
B. 52°C
C. 110°C
D. 212°C

100. Which of the following statements concerning sponges is false?

A. only radiopaque sponges should be used on the sterile field
B. sponges should be counted from the folded edge
C. a pack containing an incorrect number of sponges is discarded
D. a count is unnecessary in a vaginal procedure

101. In an extreme patient emergency a sponge count

A. may be omitted

B. may be done by the scrub alone
C. must be done before the case is allowed to begin
D. must be done before closure

102. When preparing a patient for a breast biopsy, a breast scrub is either eliminated or done very gently because of

A. patient anxiety
B. dispersal of cancer cells
C. contamination
D. infection

103. Cultures obtained during surgery

A. are handled as any other specimen
B. are passed off the sterile field into a bag or container held by the circulator
C. should be kept warm or sent to the lab immediately
D. should be handled only by the scrub nurse

104. CPR is instituted if

A. the pulse is below 60, respirations are diminished, and blood pressure is dropping
B. there is no pulse or blood pressure and the pupils contract
C. there is no pulse, respiration, or blood pressure and the pupils are fixed and dilated
D. the pulse is weak and irregular, blood pressure is lowered, and pupils are dilated

105. The ideal place to do the shave prep is in the

A. patient's room
B. OR suite
C. holding area of the OR
D. room where the surgery will be performed

106. Any area that is considered contaminated

A. should be scrubbed last or separately
B. should not be scrubbed at all
C. should be scrubbed first
D. needs no special consideration

107. In preparation for surgery, skin should be washed and painted

A. from the incision site to the periphery in a circular motion
B. from the periphery to the incision site in a circular motion
C. in a side-to-side motion
D. in an up-and-down motion

108. Preliminary preparation of the patient's skin begins

A. with a pre-op shower
B. with the shave preparation
C. in the OR
D. in the holding area

109. The main purpose of the skin prep is to

A. remove resident and transient flora
B. remove dirt, oil, and microbes and to reduce the microbial count
C. remove all bacteria from the skin
D. sterilize the patient's skin

110. Which is the antiseptic solution of choice for a skin prep?

A. Cipex
B. Staphene
C. povidone-iodine
D. Zephiran

111. When are counts done in the OR?

A. at beginning and end of case
B. before beginning of case, at beginning of wound closure, and at skin closure
C. as case begins and when case is in progress
D. before beginning a case and at end of case

112. Soiled sponges are

A. never touched with bare hands
B. left in the kick bucket until the count begins
C. removed from the room once the peritoneum is closed
D. counted and stacked on a linen towel or sheet

113. When is a pathologic specimen passed off the field?

A. as soon as the surgeon hands it to the scrub
B. never
C. at the end of the case
D. after the surgeon has granted his permission to remove it

114. When using a plastic incision drape

A. it is not necessary to paint the skin
B. the painted skin must be blotted dry before the drape is applied
C. it must be placed immediately on the moist, painted skin
D. the painted skin is allowed to air-dry before the drape is applied

115. When handling uterine curettings

A. never place them in preservative

B. keep the endometrial and the endocervical curettings separate
C. send the endometrial and the endocervical curettings to the lab in one container
D. send them on a four-by-four to the lab since it is too difficult to remove them

116. How is a frozen section sent to the lab?

A. in formalin
B. in saline
C. in water
D. dry

117. When using a sterile syringe the scrub nurse should

A. always let the surgeon attach the needle
B. always use a Luer-Lok tip
C. never use a Luer-Slip (plain) tip
D. never touch the plunger except at the end

118. Which of the following specimens is *not* placed in preservative solution?

A. stones
B. curettings
C. tonsils
D. uterus

119. The inner packet from needles should be

A. retained by the circulating nurse until the end of the case
B. retained by the scrub nurse until a final count is verified
C. discarded into the kick bucket or waste receptacle
D. placed in the same area as the discarded sponges

120. Which is the *least* desirable method of needle accountability?

A. insert needle into original packet and fold over
B. accumulate needles in a medicine cup
C. use a sterile adhesive pad, with or without a magnet, on which to store a prescribed number of needles
D. return used needles to a needle rack, or thread into the top layer of the suture book

121. Colorless prep solution may be indicated for

A. orthopedic surgery
B. vascular surgery
C. plastic surgery
D. urologic surgery

122. The universal blood donor type is _____, and the universal recipient is _____.

A. O, AB
B. O, B
C. AB, O
D. AB, A

123. An artificial plasma-volume expander is

A. mannitol
B. dextran
C. Ringer's solution
D. uromatic

124. To what does the term Rule of Nines refer?

A. fluid balance estimation
B. malpractice coverage
C. environmental ratings
D. burn classification

125. In which burn classification are the skin and subcutaneous tissue destroyed?

A. first
B. second
C. third
D. fourth

126. How many liters per minute are utilized for oxygen administration?

A. 1–2
B. 2–3
C. 6–10
D. 15–20

127. A device used to correct and counteract internal bleeding conditions and hypovolemia is a/an

A. CAT
B. IPB
C. CVP
D. MAST

128. When is a tourniquet utilized?

A. only in lower extremity bleeding
B. only when hemorrhage is not controlled by other methods
C. in all venous bleeding
D. in all arterial bleeding

129. What drug is utilized in an anaphylactic reaction?

A. atropine
B. aminophylline
C. Azo Gantrisin
D. Adrenalin

130. The patient with a suspected spinal cord injury should be placed

A. on his side
B. on a flat, hard surface with the head immobilized
C. in prone position
D. in semi-Fowler's position

131. Which position is used when caring for the patient with a suspected craniocerebral injury?

A. prone or semiprone
B. supine
C. Trendelenburg
D. reverse Trendelenburg

132. The condition in which air enters the pleural cavity, producing displacement of the heart and mediastinum with resultant cardiorespiratory embarrassment, is

A. flail chest
B. hemothorax
C. tension pneumothorax
D. pleural effusion

133. The condition of the chest wall in which it moves in with respiration and out during expiration is called

A. tension pneumothorax
B. emphysema
C. Cheyne-Stokes syndrome
D. flail chest

134. When catheterizing a patient

A. the patient must be shaved
B. the tip of the catheter must be kept sterile
C. sterile technique is not necessary
D. bag must be maintained above table level

135. To control bleeding in the arm, pressure is applied to the

A. carotid artery
B. brachial artery
C. facial artery
D. temporal artery

136. Placement of a Levin tube would be in the

A. ear
B. large intestine
C. stomach
D. bladder

137. Atelectasis is a/an

A. overdistention of lung tissue
B. pulmonary infection
C. collection of air in the pleural cavity
D. collapsed condition of the lung

138. In shock position, the patient is placed with

A. head elevated, knees flexed
B. trunk level or tilted downward about 45 degrees toward the head, legs elevated
C. head elevated higher than feet
D. head elevated, legs elevated

139. Which term indicates low or decreased blood volume?

A. anoxemia
B. hypovolemia
C. hypoxia
D. hypocapnia

E. MEDICAL/LEGAL

140. A patient was burned on the lip with a hot mouth gag. Which of the following actions would have prevented this incident?

A. the circulator cooled the item in the sterilizer
B. the scrub nurse warned the surgeon that the item was hot
C. the scrub nurse cooled the item in a basin with sterile water
D. the surgeon had checked the item before using it

141. The most effective and efficient procedure for sponge counts is to have them counted by

A. one person two times
B. two persons two times
C. one person three times
D. two persons three or more times

142. Grace F. signs a permission form for surgery, but because of a language barrier she does not fully understand what she has signed. This could constitute a liability case for

A. assault and battery
B. lack of accountability
C. improper documentation
D. invasion of privacy

143. Who is ultimately responsible for checking that the patient has removed valuables and prostheses?

A. the floor nurse
B. the circulating nurse
C. the anesthesiologist
D. the unit manager

144. An OR hazard that has been linked to increased risk of spontaneous abortion in female OR employees is exposure to

A. x-ray control
B. radium
C. sterilization agents
D. waste anesthetic gas

145. If a patient falls because he or she was left unattended, the OR team member could be sited in a lawsuit for

A. misconduct
B. assault
C. doctrine of *Respondeat Superior*
D. abandonment

146. The ultimate responsibility for obtaining consent lies with the

A. unit nurse
B. circulating nurse
C. surgeon
D. anesthesiologist

147. Which is *not* considered a safe procedure when caring for dentures inadvertently sent to the OR?

A. place in a properly labeled container
B. place in a properly labeled denture cup
C. return to the patient unit immediately and obtain a receipt, which is placed on the chart
D. wrap in a plastic bag and attach to the patient's chart

148. A lack of care or skill that any nurse or technician in the same situation would be expected to use is the legal definition of

A. assault
B. abandonment
C. negligence
D. default

149. The legal doctrine that mandates every professional nurse and technician to carry out their duties according to national standards of care practiced throughout the country is the

A. doctrine of *Res ipsa Loquitor*
B. doctrine of *Respondeat Superior*
C. Nurse Practice Act
D. doctrine of Reasonable Man

150. The doctrine of *Respondeat Superior* refers to

A. the legal terms for assault and battery
B. invasion of privacy
C. employer liability for employee's negligent conduct
D. professional misconduct

151. Liability is a legal rule that

    A. applies only in criminal actions
    B. holds the hospital responsible for its personnel
    C. holds each individual responsible for his or her own acts
    D. has no significance in malpractice suits

152. What would *never* be done on any patient having facial surgery?

    A. shave face
    B. shave eyebrows
    C. use skin prep solution
    D. use disposable razor

153. The first action to be taken in the event of a cardiac arrest in the OR is to

    A. alert the OR supervisor and personnel
    B. prepare medications
    C. institute chest massage
    D. apply fibrillator paddles

Answers and Explanations

A. PRE-OP ROUTINE

1. **(C)** Specific gravity measures the density of particles in the urine, thus showing the concentrating or diluting powers of the kidneys. The normal range is from 1.010 to 1.025. A low specific gravity (under 1.010) may indicate poor renal function, with the kidneys unable to concentrate urine. A high specific gravity (over 1.025) may indicate a dehydrated state.
   (7:897; 25:54; 36:1815)

2. **(B)** A type and cross-match of blood is done if the surgeon anticipates that blood loss replacement may be necessary. In emergency situations a sample of blood may be sent from the OR for immediate typing and cross-matching. *(2:27)*

3. **(A)** The normal range hematocrit reading in males is between 40 and 52%; in females it is between 37 and 47% of whole blood volume. Hematocrit is the percentage of blood made up of RBCs. *(36:738)*

4. **(C)** The cross-matching procedure consists of mixing a suspension of red blood cells from the donor with a small amount of defibrinated serum from the recipient. A suspension of the recipient's red cells is then mixed with donor serum. If no agglutination occurs in either case, the blood of the donor and that of the recipient are considered to be compatible, and the donor blood can be used for the transfusion.
   (34:357)

5. **(D)** A prothrombin time is clotting time test used to judge the effect of administration of anticoagulant drugs. It determines the time for clotting to occur after thromboplastin and calcium are added to decalcified plasma. *(36:1395)*

6. **(D)** Even though chest disease is not related to the patient's surgery, most surgeons consider a chest x-ray an important part of a pre-op preparation. The x-ray rules out unsuspected pulmonary disease that could be communicable or would contraindicate the use of inhalation anesthetics. *(2:290)*

7. **(A)** Electrocardiogram (ECG) is a graph of the electrical activity of the heart made with an ECG machine.
   (36:271)

8. **(B)** The hemoglobin concentration in the blood establishes the presence or absence of anemia (if low) or of polycythemia (if high). Values less than 14 g/100 ml in an adult male or less than 12 g/100 ml in an adult female would indicate anemia. A count above 18 g in either sex would indicate polycythemia. Surgery would be delayed, as bleeding is expected in tonsil surgery.
   (7:666; 36:746; 38:437, 451)

9. **(C)** In a differential blood count, the varieties of leukocytes and their percentages are estimated. It is a microscopic exam of a very thin layer of blood on a glass slide that has been stained. The normal percentages should be: neutrophils, 40 to 60%; eosinophils, 1 to 3%; basophils, 0 to 1%; lymphocytes, 20 to 40%; and monocytes, 4 to 8%. *(36:212)*

10. **(C)** Proteinuria (albuminuria) is seen characteristically in acute and chronic renal disease. Normal urine does not have protein in significant quantities. Proteinuria occurs in systemic diseases, also where there are varying degrees of renal anoxia, etc. *(7:907)*

11. **(C)** A bacteria count that is 10,000 organisms per ml of urine indicates a urinary tract infection. Bacteriuria refers to presence of bacteria in urine. *(7:937–938)*

12. **(A)** The normal pH is 6 (acid) and may vary from 4.6 to 7.5. The pH reflects the ability of the kidney to maintain normal hydrogen ion concentration in plasma and extracellular fluid. The values indicate acidity or alkalinity. *(7:907)*

13. **(B)** The SMA is a blood chemistry test providing 12 or more tests per minute. It is used to evaluate disorders that may involve such vital organs as the heart, kidneys, liver, and pancreas. It yields electrolyte and enzyme determinations, as well as glucose, urea, cholesterol, and triglyceride evaluations.   *(27:131)*

14. **(D)** The circulating nurse and anesthesiologist always check the label identifying the patient and surgeon; they also check the patient's chart and the operating schedule. The surgeon sees the patient before anesthetic agents are administered.   *(2:508)*

15. **(D)** In a dire emergency, the patient's condition takes precedence over the permit. Permits may be accepted from a legal guardian or responsible relative. Two nurses should monitor a phone consent and sign the form; it is then signed by the parent, guardian, or spouse upon arrival. A written consultation by two physicians, not including the surgeon, will suffice until the proper signature can be obtained.   *(2:45)*

16. **(C)** An informed consent or operative permit is a written, properly witnessed permission which protects the patient against unsanctioned surgery and protects the surgeon and the hospital against claims of unauthorized operations. Before signing, the patient should be told what the surgeon will do. The surgeon should also explain possible complications, disfigurement, and disability as well as what post-op expectations are.   *(7:311)*

17. **(C)** If the surgeon intends or wants to perform a procedure not specified on the permission or consent form, the OR nurse assumes the responsibility of informing the surgeon and/or the proper administrative authority of the discrepancy.   *(2:45)*

18. **(D)** The patient's (or suitable substitute's) signature must be witnessed by one or more authorized persons. They may be physicians, nurses, or other hospital employees authorized to do so. The witness is attesting to the proper identification of the patient and the fact that the signing was voluntary.   *(2:45)*

19. **(A)** The patient giving his consent must be of legal age, mentally alert, and competent. The patient must sign before premedication is given and before going to the OR. This protects the patient from unratified procedures as well as protecting the surgeon and the hospital.   *(2:45)*

20. **(A)** The general consent form authorizes the physician in charge and hospital staff to render such treatments or perform such procedures as the physician deems advisable. It applies only to routine hospital procedures. The consent document for any procedure possibly injurious to the patient should be signed before the procedure is performed.   *(2:44)*

21. **(C)** The ultimate responsibility for obtaining permission is the surgeon's. The circulating nurse (RN or charge) and the anesthesiologist are responsible for checking that the consent is on the chart, properly signed, and that the information on the form is correct.   *(2:45)*

22. **(D)** This is a real fear and cannot be dismissed lightly. Good rapport and tact between patient and nurse may bring patient to the realization that his or her fear is magnified.   *(7:308)*

23. **(A)** Unfulfilled spiritual needs can cause patient anxiety. The spiritual advisory should be permitted to see the patient before he undergoes surgery.   *(2:34)*

24. **(D)** Adipose tissue retains anesthetic drugs longer because many of the drugs are fat soluble and the tissue has poor blood supply. Healing may be delayed because of poor vascularity. There is an increased incidence of wound infection and disruption.   *(2:61)*

25. **(C)** Oral intake is discontinued, usually the patient is NPO (nothing by mouth) for 8 hours preceding operation. This is done to prevent regurgitation or emesis and aspiration of contents. The preoperative medication contains an anticholinergic for inhibition of mucous secretions. The patient usually complains of dry mouth after their administration.   *(2:65, 165)*

26. **(B)** A myelogram is an x-ray of the spinal canal after injection of a radiopaque dye into the intrathecal space. It is carried out with a water-soluble contrast media mostly via a lumbar puncture. It is used as a diagnostic study.   *(36:1085)*

27. **(D)** All consent forms must be signed before the administration of pre-op medications. This is to ensure that the patient fully understands what the procedure is. If the permission is signed incorrectly, it may not be revised until the pre-op medication has worn off.   *(32:29)*

28. **(B)** pH measures degree of acidity or alkalinity of a substance. The normal pH of blood is 7.35 to 7.45. The neutral point where a solution would be neither acid or alkaline is pH 7. Increasing acidity is expressed in a number less than 7 and increasing alkalinity as a number greater than 7.   *(36:210, 1277)*

29. **(A)** A bowel preparation for intestinal surgery is mechanical (diet, enema, laxatives) and chemical (antibiotics) in an attempt to eliminate pathogenic bacteria.   *(32:210; 36:462, 549, 935)*

B. TRANSPORTATION

30. **(C)** Four people are needed to move the patient safely when using a roller. One lifts the head, one lifts the feet, one is beside the stretcher, and one is beside the OR table. *(2:149)*

31. **(C)** Weights are never removed from a patient with a fracture unless a life-threatening situation occurs. They should be supported and prevented from swinging as pulling creates an opposite reaction from the intended force. *(7:1289)*

32. **(C)** It is the responsibility of the anesthesiologist to guard the neck and head. It also puts him in a better position to observe the patient. Four people are needed and the action must be synchronized. *(2:149)*

33. **(B)** There should be an adequate number of personnel to safely transfer the patient to the OR table. One person should stand next to the stretcher to stabilize it against the adjacent OR table. Another receives the patient from the opposite side of the table. If a patient is unable to help move himself, additional people are necessary. *(11:288)*

34. **(D)** Transport stretchers should be equipped with side rails, restraining strap, IV pole, and brakes. This ensures patient safety. *(11:288)*

35. **(B)** Fractures should be handled gently. Support should be both above and below the fracture site when moving the patient. Adequate personnel should be available. The lifters on the affected side support the fracture site. *(2:372)*

36. **(B)** Personnel who transport the patient should be courteous and gentle. The patient may become anxious if the personnel act as though they are in a hurry. Consistent, deliberate movements are appreciated by the patient. *(5:23)*

37. **(C)** Occult blood is blood in such a minute quantity that it can be recognized only by a microscopic exam or chemical means. *(36:1152)*

38. **(D)** The patient's bed may be used in place of a stretcher if his or her condition requires as little movement as possible. This would be true for critically ill patients or patients with fractures. *(5:23)*

39. **(C)** The safety strap should be applied securely but loosely about 2 inches above the knee. This is to avoid compromise of venous circulation or pressure on bony prominences or nerves. *(2:144; 32:92)*

40. **(B)** The physician is responsible for supporting and protecting the fracture site when moving the orthopedic patient. A fracture is handled gently with support above and below the fracture site. *(2:372)*

C. POSITIONING

41. **(D)** Patient's arms should not be crossed on the chest in order to prevent hindrance of diaphragmatic movement and airway. This is essential to maintain respiratory function, to prevent hypoxia, and to facilitate inhalation anesthesia induction. *(2:212)*

42. **(C)** Trendelenburg position is used for procedures in the lower abdomen or pelvis in which it is desirable to tilt the abdominal viscera away from the pelvic area for better exposure. The entire table is tilted downward (about 45 degrees at the head) while the foot is also lowered the desired amount. *(2:216)*

43. **(D)** In the supine position, heels must be protected from pressure on the table by a pillow, ankle roll, or doughnut. The feet must not be in prolonged flexion, the soles are supported to prevent footdrop. *(2:215)*

44. **(B)** Femoral nerve injury could be the result of careless retractor use during pelvic surgery. Retractors should be well padded to protect nerves. Assistants should not pull too hard on them. *(2:212)*

45. **(D)** Good respiratory function begins with unfastening of the patient's gown before anesthesia begins so that there is no constriction on the throat. *(5:97)*

46. **(A)** The buttocks should be even with the table edge but should not extend over the edge; otherwise it could cause strain to the lumbosacral muscles and ligaments, since the body weight rests on the sacrum. *(2:217)*

47. **(A)** The anesthesia screen is placed after induction and positioning of the patient. It is placed after induction and positioning so that these efforts are not impeded. *(2:213)*

48. **(D)** Legs are raised simultaneously by two people who grasp the sole of a foot in one hand and support the knee area with the other. Stirrups must be of equal height and appropriate for size of patient's leg. *(2:217)*

49. **(B)** The Kraske (jackknife) position is used for procedures in the rectal area such as pilonidal sinus or hemorrhoidectomy. Feet and toes are protected by a pillow. The head is to the side and the arms are on armboards. *(2:218)*

50. **(A)** In the Fowler's position the patient lies on his or her back with knees over the lower break in the table. A footboard is raised and padded. The foot of the table is lowered slightly, flexing the knees. The body section is raised. Arms rest on a pillow on the lap. This position is used in some cranial procedures with the head supported in a headrest. *(2:217)*

51. **(D)** The Kraske position is also called the jackknife position. Patient is anesthetized in supine position. He or she is turned to abdomen with the hips over center break in the table.   *(2:218)*

52. **(A)** The OR table is flexed so that the kidney elevator can be raised the desired amount to increase the space between lower ribs and iliac crest. A body strap or tape is placed over the hips. The safety belt is over the legs.   *(2:219)*

53. **(A)** When the patient is in prone position, the safety strap is placed below the knees. A pillow under the ankles and feet prevents pressure on the toes.   *(2:218)*

54. **(B)** The patient is in prone position with lumbar spine over the center break of the table; two laminectomy rolls (or other firm padding) are placed longitudinally to support the chest from axilla to hip. Additional padding protects bony prominences.   *(20:130)*

55. **(B)** When the kidney position is being used, the table is straightened before closure to afford better approximation of tissues. It is used for procedures on kidneys and ureters. This is done by the anesthesiologist.   *(2:219)*

56. **(D)** The requirements of the Kraske position are: patient is prone with hips over break of table, wide armboard is under head of mattress to support arms, pillow is under lower legs and ankles, padded knee strap is 2 inches above knees, table is flexed to acute angle, and small rolled towel is under each shoulder.   *(20:128)*

57. **(B)** The anesthesiologist must give his permission before the patient is moved. This is a safety measure as his readiness to direct the move is important.   *(2:212)*

58. **(C)** Placement of the patient in the operative position is the responsibility of the circulating nurse with the guidance, approval, and sometimes assistance of the surgeon and the anesthesiologist. It is a shared responsibility. If the circulator needs help, she should request it.   *(2:211)*

59. **(C)** When using an armboard, caution should be taken so that the arm is not hyperextended or the infusion needle dislodged. Hyperextension can cause nerve damage.   *(2:211–212)*

60. **(D)** The anesthetized patient and the elderly patient must be moved slowly and gently. This allows the circulatory system to adjust. This is for patient safety.   *(2:212)*

61. **(C)** The patient must not have ankles or legs crossed as this could create pressure on blood vessels and nerves. A normal reaction is for a supine patient to cross his or her legs before going to sleep.   *(2:12)*

62. **(D)** Injury to the brachial plexus can result from extreme positions of the head and arm. This can be avoided with proper care and careful observation.   *(2:12)*

63. **(D)** Ulnar nerve damage can occur from pressure from the OR table edge. The arm resting on an unpadded surface places pressure on the ulnar nerve as it transverses the elbow. This can be prevented by the use of padding, by fastening the arm securely with a lift sheet, or by placing the arms on armboards.   *(11:77)*

64. **(A)** A modified Trendelenburg position is used for patients in hypovolemic shock. This may aid in venous return and cardiac output.   *(2:201, 217)*

65. **(A)** The thorax is elevated when the patient is in prone position in order to facilitate respiration. This is accomplished with supports, rolls, elevating pads, body rests, or braces.   *(2:212–214)*

66. **(B)** The patient's eyes may remain open even when the patient is under anesthesia. This exposes them to drying or trauma from drapes or instruments. They can be protected with ophthalmic ointment or taped closed.   *(11:79)*

D. RELATED NURSING PROCEDURES

67. **(C)** The scrub nurse and the circulator count each item aloud and together. The nurse then records the number. Count additional items away from already counted items. Counting should be uninterrupted.   *(2:150)*

68. **(A)** When a cardiac arrest occurs in the OR, the anesthesiologist handles the artificial respiration. He may already have an endotracheal tube in place or an airway.   *(2:205)*

69. **(A)** Pulmonary embolus is an obstruction of one or more of the pulmonary arteries by a thrombus that becomes dislodged and is carried to the lung. This may be accompanied by sudden substernal pain, rapid and weak pulse, shock, syncope, and sudden death. It is often associated with advanced age and postoperative states.   *(7:490–491)*

70. **(A)** If a pack contains an incorrect number of sponges, it is the responsibility of the circulator to take it from the scrub and remove it from the room immediately. The danger of error is great if attempts are made to correct or compensate for discrepancies.   *(2:251)*

71. **(A)** Each item used must be considered a foreign object that can cause unnecessary harm should it be left inside the patient. Detachable parts of instruments must be counted. This assures that part of an instrument does not remain in the wound.   *(2:150–151)*

72. **(A)** Suprapubic bladder drainage is drainage of the bladder through a percutaneous puncture or open incision into the bladder. It is indicated following urethral injuries, when a sterile urine sample is needed, following a vaginal hysterectomy and vaginal repair operation, and after prostatic surgery.   *(7:913–914)*

73. **(C)** Sponges should be kept away from linen, instruments, and needles. Sponges and tapes should not be in a basin at the same time because a small sponge may be dragged unknowingly into the wound along with a tape. Keep a mental count of the number of sponges on the field.   *(2:152)*

74. **(C)** Amputated extremities are wrapped before sending them to a refrigerator. The morgue is the usual place that receives them unless hospital policy dictates otherwise. They must be tagged and labeled properly.   *(2:148)*

75. **(B)** The carotid pulse is palpated in CPR. The carotid arises from the aorta. It is the principal blood supply to the head and neck and is palpable in the neck.   *(2:204; 36:274)*

76. **(B)** Diastolic blood pressure is that which exists during the relaxation phase between heartbeats. It is the point at which sound is no longer heard. Normal is about 80.   *(36:213)*

77. **(D)** Systolic blood pressure occurs when a great force is caused by contraction of the left ventricle of the heart. The first sound heard is recorded as the systolic pressure.   *(36:214)*

78. **(D)** Hypothermia is body temperature below normal. Hypothermia is a technique to lower body temperature to 78 to 90°F. This reduces oxygen needs especially during cardiac, vascular, or neurosurgery.   *(36:813)*

79. **(C)** Often the anesthesiologist leaves a hard rubber or plastic airway in the mouth. This should remain in place until the patient recovers sufficiently to breathe normally. It should not be removed until the patient expresses a desire to have it removed.   *(7:348)*

80. **(D)** Malignant hyperthermia is an often fatal complication characterized by progressive elevation of the body temperature monitored as high as 109°F. It occurs most often during general anesthesia and its exact cause is unknown. If untreated it can result in cardiovascular collapse.   *(2:198)*

81. **(C)** Lidocaine is used where successful defibrillation reverts back repeatedly to ventricular fibrillation. The trade name is Xylocaine.   *(2:208)*

82. **(A)** Tachycardia is excessive rapidity of heart action. The pulse rate is over 100 beats per minute. Some of the most common causes are exercise, anxiety, fever, and shock.   *(2:163; 7:527)*

83. **(C)** The normal pulse rate in a healthy athletic person may vary from a low of 50 to rates well in excess of 100 following exercise. Bradycardia is seen normally in well-trained athletes.   *(7:527)*

84. **(B)** The pulse deficit is the difference between the apical pulse rate (taken at the apex of the heart) and the peripheral pulse rate (taken at a distal vessel such as the radial artery of the wrist). A deficit often occurs during serious heart disease.   *(7:68)*

85. **(D)** The true configuration of the pulse is best taken by palpating the carotid artery rather than a distal artery, because the pulse wave may be distorted by transmission to smaller vessels. The examiner must also be aware of occluded vessels characterized by absence of pulsation.   *(7:68)*

86. **(A)** Without the patient's knowledge (if possible), count each inspiration and expiration as one breath. Watch the rise and fall of the chest and upper abdomen for 1 full minute. Breathing is both voluntary and involuntary.   *(36:1476)*

87. **(C)** The telethermometer monitors the body temperature during an operation. It is electronic, connects to a probe, and provides direct temperature readouts on a dial. Rectal, esophageal, or tympanic probes are used. This is frequently used in pediatric surgery.   *(2:459)*

88. **(D)** Hypoxia is lack of adequate amounts of oxygen; if prolonged, it can result in cardiac arrhythmia or irreversible brain, liver, kidney, and heart damage. The treatment is immediate adequate oxygen intake to stimulate the medullary centers and prevent respiratory system failure. Dark blood on the operative field is a symptom of hypoxia.   *(2:197)*

89. **(C)** Immediate opening of the airway is the most important factor for successful resuscitation. The back of the tongue is the most common obstruction. Since the tongue is attached to the lower jaw, moving the jaw forward lifts the tongue from the back of the throat and opens the airway.   *(1:19)*

90. **(D)** The scrub nurse should pay attention to the field and the surgeon's needs. Scrub nurses should also keep syringes of medications filled and ready for use, keep track of sponges, and be prepared to close the wound rapidly. If arrest occurs during the operation, the wound is packed and the patient repositioned for CPR. *(2:209)*

91. **(A)** Morphine is an analgesic which also treats acute pulmonary edema. Morphine pools blood peripherally and decreases venous return. In doing so, it assists in relieving pulmonary congestion and decreases myocardial oxygen requirements. *(2:208)*

92. **(D)** Atropine sulfate is most useful in preventing arrest in profound sinus bradycardia secondary to myocardial infarct, particularly when hypotension is present. The dose is 0.5 to 1 mg. Atropine inhibits the vagal nerve thus makes heart go faster. *(7:528)*

93. **(A)** When using the defibrillator, neither the person holding the electrodes nor anyone else may touch the patient or anything metallic that is in contact with the patient. This is done to prevent self-electrocution. No part of the operator's body should touch the paste or insulated electrodes. *(2:202)*

94. **(C)** External, cardiac compression maintains circulation, which provides oxygen to vital body tissues and keeps them viable. It also preserves cardiac tone and reflexes and prevents intravascular clotting. It is the rhythmic application of pressure which compresses the ventricles. *(2:205–206)*

95. **(D)** When handing a syringe with a local anesthetic to the surgeon, the scrub nurse should state the kind and percentage of the solution. This action prevents errors. *(2:139)*

96. **(A)** The solution label on a local infiltrative anesthetic is checked by a registered nurse when it is poured and verified when it is given. The scrub nurse states the kind and percentage of the solution when handing the syringe to the surgeon. *(2:139)*

97. **(B)** Resuscitative measures must be instituted immediately (within 3 to 5 minutes to prevent irreversible brain damage. Time of arrest should be noted. A clock should be started to check time lapse. *(2:204)*

98. **(B)** It is the circulating nurse's responsibility to keep a record of all medications given, including the time and the amount. One person, usually the anesthesiologist, commands the effort with support from others. *(2:209)*

99. **(A)** To convert Farenheit to Celsius, subtract 32 from the number of Farenheit degrees and multiply the difference by 5/9, as

$$98.6°F - 32.0 = 66.6, \text{ times } 5/9 = 37°C$$

(36:1905)

100. **(D)** Sponge and instrument counts are very important in vaginal procedures. Sponges should be secured on sticks in deep areas. This prevents loss in hard to see areas. *(2:238)*

101. **(A)** Omitted counts due to extreme patient emergency must be documented on the operative record and a patient incident report completed by the circulating nurse. This is only acceptable in a life-threatening emergency. *(2:151)*

102. **(B)** When a breast is prepped for suspected malignancy, it is done gently or eliminated. Scrubbing the breast with the usual amount of pressure could cause cancer cells to break loose from the lesion and spread the disease. *(17:82)*

103. **(B)** Cultures are obtained under sterile conditions. The tips must not be contaminated by any other source. The circulating nurse can hold open a small bag for the scrub nurse to drop the tube into if it is handled on the sterile field. This protects personnel and prevents the spread of microorganisms. *(2:147–148)*

104. **(C)** The patient is in cardiopulmonary arrest if there is no pulse, respiration, or blood pressure and the pupils are dilated. If unconscious, check airway; if not breathing, resuscitation; if no pulse and pupils are dilated, massage heart. *(36:272)*

105. **(C)** The patient should be shaved immediately prior to surgery, preferably in a holding area of the OR; this is thought to reduce the infection rate. The amount of time between the preoperative shave and the operation has a direct effect on wound infection rate. *(32:66)*

106. **(A)** Contaminated areas (which can include draining sinuses, skin ulcers, vagina, or anus) should be scrubbed last or with separate sponges. This prevents dragging pathogens into the incisional area and thus reduces the possibility of infection. *(2:225)*

107. **(A)** Skin should be washed from the incision site to the periphery in a circular motion. This keeps the incision site cleaner and prevents wound contamination. *(2:224)*

108. **(A)** Patients may be advised to begin bathing with a 3% hexachlorophene solution before admission for an elective procedure. Patients should shower or be bathed before coming to the OR suite. This action is bacteriostatic and reduces microbial contamination. *(2:222)*

109. **(B)** Methods of skin prep may vary but the objectives are the same: to remove dirt, oil, and microbes from the skin so the incision can be made through the skin with a minimal danger of infection. It also reduces resident microbial count and prevents the growth of microbes. *(32:64)*

110. **(C)** The current trend is toward a surgical scrub of antiseptic solution containing povidine-iodine. This reduces the number of bacteria on the skin and inhibits the growth. This process is eliminated in some ORs. *(11:253)*

111. **(B)** The first count is done by the instrument wrapper at assembly. The second count is immediately before the operation begins by the scrub and the circulator. A third count is done when wound closure is started. A fourth is done for any discrepancy and at skin closure. An additional count may be done when a cavity within a cavity is closed, e.g., uterus. *(2:150–151)*

112. **(A)** Soiled sponges should never be touched with bare hands. Sponges should be counted in units and bagged in waterproof plastic bag or transferred to a moisture-proof surface until the final count is completed. This is done to avoid hepatitis or pathogenic organism transmission. *(2:152)*

113. **(D)** A specimen can be passed off to the circulator *only* after the surgeon has granted permission for its removal from the sterile field. This is to assure that all tissue has been removed that the surgeon wants as specimen or that all contaminated items are in the specimen basin. *(2:141; 17:197)*

114. **(B)** When a plastic incision drape is used, the painted skin must be blotted dry so that the drape will adhere to the skin. The scrub should provide a sterile towel for this. *(23:57)*

115. **(B)** The endometrial curettings should be kept separate from the endocervical curettings. Fractional curettage specimens differentiate between the endocervical and the endometrium of the corpus which helps to locate a lesion more specifically. *(2:345–346)*

116. **(D)** Frozen section specimens are not placed in solution as it can react with tissue and affect the pathologist's diagnosis. A frozen section is the cutting of a thin piece of tissue from a frozen specimen. This permits examination under a microscope. *(17:198; 36:649)*

117. **(D)** The scrub nurse should not touch the plunger except at the end, because glove powder can act as a contaminant. Contamination of the plunger can contaminate the inner wall of the barrel and the solution that is drawn into it. *(2:139)*

118. **(A)** Stones are placed in a dry container to prevent dissolving. Stones are sent for additional study to determine their composition. *(2:148)*

119. **(B)** The scrub nurse retains the inner descriptive needle or needled suture packet in order to help determine whether the count is correct for swaged and disposable needles. They should not be discarded until after case completion and verification of correct final count. *(2:151)*

120. **(B)** Needles are not safely stored in a medicine cup because of difficulty in counting them and the chance of puncturing the glove when removing them. Also by handling each needle individually, the potential for contamination increases. *(2:153)*

121. **(C)** A colorless prep solution may be used in plastic surgery to facilitate observation of the true color of the skin. *(2:444)*

122. **(A)** The universal donor is O. The universal recipient is AB. Individuals whose erythrocytes manufacture only agglutinogen have type A blood. Those who only manufacture agglutinogen B are type B. Individuals who manufacture both A and B are type AB. Those who manufacture neither are type O. *(38:447–449)*

123. **(B)** Dextran is an artificial volume expander which acts by drawing the fluid from the tissues. It remains in the circulation for several hours. It is used in emergency situations to treat shock by increasing blood volume. *(2:144)*

124. **(D)** The Rule of Nines is a method used to estimate the total percentage of body surface burned and the percentage of each degree of burn. The body surface is divided into areas equal to multiples of 9 percent of the total body surface. *(2:453)*

125. **(C)** In a third-degree burn the skin with all its epithelial structures and subcutaneous tissue are destroyed. These burns require skin graft for healing to occur. *(2:453)*

126. **(B)** Oxygen is administered according to patient's needs using nasal prongs at 6 liters per minute or by face mask at 10 liters per minute. Patient should be observed for signs of anoxia. *(19:356–357)*

127. **(D)** The Medical Anti-Shock Trouser (MAST) is a garment designed to correct and counteract internal bleeding conditions and hypovolemia. It creates an encircling pressure around both legs and abdomen. It slows or stops arterial bleeding, forces any available blood from the lower body to the heart, brain, and other vital organs, and it prevents the return of available circulating blood volume to the lower extremities. *(7:1420)*

128. **(B)** Apply a tourniquet only as a last resort when hemorrhage cannot be controlled by any other means. Tourniquets can cause irreparable vascular or neurologic damage. *(7:1419)*

129. **(D)** Anaphylaxis is a generalized systemic and frequently fatal reaction occuring within minutes after administration of foreign sera or drugs. Epinephrine chloride is given. This provides rapid relief or hypersensitivity reaction. This is also called adrenalin. *(7:1429)*

130. **(B)** The patient is kept on a flat, hard stretcher or board with the head immobilized. The spine should not be moved and the back should be kept straight since flexion or extension can increase the cord injury. The head, legs, knees, and arms should also be kept straight. *(7:1253)*

131. **(A)** The patient with a head injury is kept prone or semiprone after making certain there is no cervical spine injury. The prone position facilitates drainage from the tracheobronchial tree and minimizes aspiration of nasopharyngeal and gastric secretions. It also decreases intracranial pressure. *(7:1192–1193; 1249)*

132. **(C)** Tension pneumothorax occurs when air enters the pleural cavity, producing displacement of the heart and mediastinum to the uninvolved side, with resultant severe cardiorespiratory embarrassment. This may be caused by penetration of the chest wall, laceration or perforation of the lung by in-driven fractured ribs, or alveolar rupture from blunt trauma. *(7:499)*

133. **(D)** Flail chest is the condition of the chest wall when, due to multiple fractures of the rib cage, it moves paradoxically in with inspiration and out during expiration. This impairs the ability to produce negative intrapleural pressure required to draw in air. Severe flail is treated by a tracheotomy. *(7:498)*

134. **(B)** Urinary catheterization requires sterile technique as contamination can lead to urinary tract infection. The drainage bag is always maintained below the table level. This prevents contamination by retrograde or backward flow of urine. *(2:221)*

135. **(B)** Pressure on the brachial artery helps to stop bleeding in the arm. The brachial artery is the main artery of the arm. *(36:223)*

136. **(C)** A Levin tube is a catheter which is introduced usually through the nose. It extends through the stomach into the duodenum. It is used to help prevent accumulation of intestinal liquids and gas during and following intestinal surgery. *(36:951)*

137. **(D)** When a mucous plug entirely closes one of the bronchi, there is a collapse of pulmonary tissue beyond, resulting in atelectasis (collapse of the lung or airless lung). It can also occur from pressure on the lung tissue restricting normal lung expansion. *(7:412)*

138. **(B)** Trendelenburg position – the patient lies on his back with the knees over the lower break in the table, foot of the table is lowered, flexing the knees. A modification for hypovolemic shock is trunk level and legs elevated by raising lower part of table at break under the hips. Another preference is to tilt the entire table downward about 45 degrees at the head. *(2:216–217)*

139. **(B)** Hypovolemia means low or decreased blood volume. The blood volume of an average size male is 5 to 6 liters (10 to 12 pints) and an average female 4 to 5 liters (8 to 10 pints). Hypovolemic shock is caused by a decrease in circulating blood volume from loss of blood, plasma, or extracellular fluid. It is reversed by prompt restoration of blood volume via a transfusion of whole blood or other IV fluid or plasma expander. *(2:162, 201; 17:436)*

E. MEDICAL/LEGAL

140. **(C)** It is the responsibility of the scrub nurse to cool an instrument in cool sterile water before handing it to the surgeon. Burns are one of the most frequent causes of lawsuits. *(2:509)*

141. **(D)** Sponges, needles, and instruments are counted at four different times. The first time (not part of the immediate surgery) is done by the person who wraps the items for sterilization. The next count is done by the circulating and scrub nurses before the operation begins, followed by a count when wound closure begins. A fourth count is done if a discrepancy is noted or at skin closure. *(2:150–151)*

142. **(A)** Lack of consent is an aspect of assault and battery. Consent must be given voluntarily with full understanding of the implications. The procedure must be explained fully, in understandable language, so that the patient fully comprehends what will be done. *(2:504)*

143. **(B)** The circulating nurse has the responsibility of double-checking the patient for contact lenses, dentures, artificial limbs, glass eye, wigs, rings, etc., even though they should have been removed on the unit before the patient came to the OR. *(2:508)*

144. **(D)** Waste anesthetic gas is gas and vapor that escape from the anesthesia machine and equipment, as well as gas released through the patient's expiration. The hazards to personnel include an increased risk of spon-

taneous abortion in females working in the OR, congenital abnormalities in their children as well as in the offspring of unexposed wives of exposed male personnel, cancer in females administering anesthesia, and hepatic and renal disease in both males and females. This problem can be reduced by a scavenging system which removes waste gases.   *(2:177)*

145. **(D)** Abandonment may be a cause for a lawsuit if an unattended patient falls from a stretcher or an OR table. It is the responsibility of a staff member to stay with the patient at all times.   *(2:508)*

146. **(C)** The surgeon has the ultimate responsibility for obtaining the consent. The consent document becomes a permanent part of the patient's medical record and accompanies him to the OR.   *(2:45)*

147. **(D)** The nurse should place dentures in a properly labeled container and return them immediately to the unit. He or she will obtain a receipt, which is placed on the patient's chart. The transaction is recorded in the nurse's notes.   *(2:508)*

148. **(C)** Negligence is legally defined as "the omission to do something which a reasonable person, guided by those ordinary considerations which ordinarily regulate human affairs, would do, or doing something which a reasonable and prudent person would not do."   *(2:503)*

149. **(D)** The Doctrine of Reasonable Man means that a patient has the right to expect all professional and technical nursing personnel to utilize knowledge, skill, and judgment in performing duties that meet the standards exercised by other reasonable, prudent persons involved in a similar circumstance.   *(2:503)*

150. **(C)** An employer may be liable for an employee's negligent conduct under the *Respondeat Superior* master–servant employment relationship. This implies that the master will answer for the acts of the servant.   *(2:504)*

151. **(C)** An unconditional general rule of law is that every person is liable for the wrongs he or she commits which cause injury, loss, or damage to any person's property. Liability means to be legally bound, answerable, and responsible. A patient or family member may institute a civil action against the person who caused the injury, loss, or damage.   *(2:503)*

152. **(B)** It is rarely necessary to shave the face of females or children. The eyebrows are *never* shaved, since hair tends not to grow back in scar tissue.   *(32:70)*

153. **(A)** Most hospitals are equipped with a special code switch or foot pedal that sets off an alarm indicating an arrest in the room in which it occurs. Within seconds additional personnel will be available to aid in resuscitation efforts.   *(17:203)*

CHAPTER 3

Aseptic Technique and Environmental Control
Questions

Directions: Each of the questions or incomplete statements below is followed by four suggested answers or completions. Select the best answer in each case.

A. STERILIZATION, DISINFECTION, AND ANTISEPSIS

1. The pounds of pressure necessary in a steam sterilizer set at 250°F is

A. 15
B. 17
C. 20
D. 27

2. When steam enters the steam sterilizer under pressure, it forces the heavier air ahead of it and forward until it is discharged at the front of the sterilizer. This is called

A. come-up time
B. gravity displacement
C. steam penetration time
D. exposure period

3. The most dependable control measure used to assure that sterile conditions have been achieved is

A. biologic control test
B. heat-sensitive tape
C. color change indicators
D. process monitor

4. When the steam autoclave door is opened

A. items are removed immediately
B. items are placed on a table to cool
C. items remain untouched to dry for 10 to 30 minutes
D. items are immediately moved to storage areas

5. A wrapped tray of instruments is sterilized in a gravity displacement sterilizer at 250°F for

A. 10 minutes
B. 15 minutes
C. 30 minutes
D. 40 minutes

6. The minimum exposure time for unwrapped instruments in a flash sterilizer which is set at 270°F (132°C) is

A. 2 minutes
B. 3 minutes
C. 5 minutes
D. 7 minutes

7. When steam is used to sterilize a rubber tubing or catheter

A. the lumen must be dried thoroughly before the process begins
B. a rubber band may be placed around it so it does not unwind
C. it should be fan-folded before wrapping
D. a residual of distilled water should be left inside the lumen

8. In order to be effectively sterilized, a linen pack must not weigh more than

A. 12 lb
B. 14 lb
C. 16 lb
D. 18 lb

9. The safest, most practical method for linen sterilization is

A. ETO
B. steam
C. hot air–dry heat
D. ionizing radiation

10. The necessary temperature for a high-vacuum sterilizer is

A. 250–254°F
B. 255–260°F
C. 265–270°F
D. 272–276°F

11. The washer-sterilizer utilizes

A. steam under pressure
B. dry heat
C. ionizing radiation
D. chemical agents

12. The process called cavitation occurs in the

A. moist heat sterilizer
B. ultrasonic cleaner
C. high-speed pressure sterilizer
D. washer-sterilizer

13. All of the following statements regarding instrument sets are true except

A. instruments must be placed in perforated trays
B. heavy instruments are placed on the bottom
C. all instruments must be closed
D. all detachable parts must be disassembled

14. Which statement regarding steam sterilization is false?

A. flat packages are placed on the shelf on edge
B. small packages, placed one on top of the other, are criss-crossed
C. basins are placed on their sides
D. solutions may be autoclaved along with other items as long as they are on a shelf alone

15. Wrapped basin sets may be sterilized by steam under pressure at 250°F for a minimum of

A. 5 minutes
B. 10 minutes
C. 15 minutes
D. 20 minutes

16. Which of the following statements regarding the sterilization of basin sets is true?

A. basins must be separated by a porous material if they are nested
B. sponges and linen may be packaged inside the basin to be sterilized
C. basins are placed flat in the autoclave
D. basins must always be placed on the bottom shelf of the autoclave

17. Why would gas sterilization be chosen over steam sterilization?

A. it is less expensive
B. it is less damaging to items
C. it is faster
D. it is more effective

18. Dry heat is used primarily to sterilize

A. instrument sets
B. linen packs
C. lensed instruments and tubing
D. anhydrous oils, petroleum products, and bulk powders

19. The chemical agent used in gas sterilization is

A. quaternary ammonium
B. ultraviolet irradiation
C. glutaraldehyde
D. ethylene oxide

20. The main disadvantage of ETO sterilization is

A. length of process
B. special equipment
C. skin irritant
D. aeration time

21. Which item or items require aeration time after gas sterilization?

A. glass
B. metal
C. rubber
D. all of the above

22. A common type of sterilization process utilized in the commercial preparation of products is

A. ionizing radiation
B. dry heat
C. steam sterilization
D. chemical sterilization

23. Why is ethylene oxide diluted with an inert gas such as fluorinated hydrocarbon or carbon dioxide?

A. this mixture provides a safe, nonflammable agent as EO is highly flammable and explosive by itself
B. it is not effective by itself
C. it makes EO more convenient to work with
D. this mixture adds humidity, which is a more effective medium

24. Which agent has the quality of being sporicidal?

A. formaldehyde
B. iodophor
C. alcohol
D. phenol

25. The most common agent in irradiation sterilization is

A. ultraviolet light
B. radium
C. Cidex
D. cobalt 60

26. The usual temperature in a gas sterilizer is

A. 80–100°F
B. 100–120°F
C. 120–140°F
D. 200–240°F

27. Which of the following is essential when using activated glutaraldehyde for sterilization?

A. items must be rinsed thoroughly in sterile water before use
B. the solution must be heated in order to be effective
C. the items must be thoroughly moistened before placement in solution
D. the item must be air-dried before use

28. An example of an activated glutaraldehyde is

A. alcohol (70–95%)
B. Cidex
C. iodophor
D. benzalkonium chloride

29. Which of the following is the *least* effective housekeeping disinfectant for hospital use?

A. quaternary ammonium compound
B. phenol compound
C. iodophor compound
D. alcohol

30. Which statement regarding the use of alcohol as a disinfectant is false?

A. it leaves no residue on treated surfaces
B. it is bactericidal, pseudomonicidal, and fungicidal in a minimum of 10 minutes' exposure
C. it is tuberculocidal and virucidal in a minimum of 15 minutes' exposure
D. it is recommended for lensed instruments

31. Spore formation occurs within the cell. This growth can be referred to as

A. endodermic
B. endoplastic
C. endometric
D. endogenic

32. A disinfectant solution with a phenol detergent base is

A. alcohol
B. Zephirin
C. Staphene
D. Wescodyne

33. In order to kill spores, an item must be immersed in a 2% aqueous solution of glutaraldehyde for

A. 20 minutes
B. 2 hours
C. 10 hours
D. 24 hours

34. Activa
10 minut

A. bact
B. tub
C. sp
D. vi

35.
glu

A.
B. be cer
completely fillec
C. moisten it thoroughly be
D. B and C

36. What is the role of moisture in EO sterilization?

A. the items will dry out during the process if no humidity is added
B. the sterilizer will deteriorate from gas over a period of time if no moisture is added
C. dried spores are resistant to the gas, so they must be hydrated
D. moisture is not an essential element in gas sterilization

37. The minimum exposure time in a conventional steam sterilizer is

A. 5 minutes
B. 10 minutes
C. 15 minutes
D. 30 minutes

38. Sterilizer-indicating tape used on the outside of a package indicates absolutely that

A. a package is sterile
B. a package has been exposed to the physical conditions of the sterilization cycle
C. a package was sterile
D. the sterilizer is working satisfactorily

39. What is the function of an aerator in EO sterilization?

A. it is used to aerate items before sterilization
B. it is a separate unit used to decrease the aeration time
C. it is the last cycle in the EO sterilizer which helps exhaust the gas and add air
D. it adds air to the cycle, which is essential for obtaining item sterility

40. Ethylene oxide
interfering w
protein an
A.
B. coagulati
C. conver
causi
D. shr

41.

destroys cells by

th the normal metabolism of the
reproductive processes
ng cell protein
ng ions to thermal and chemical energy
ng cell death
nking the cell

For adequate steam sterilization items must be

A. dry
B. wet
C. free of grease and oil
D. processed in cavitron

B. PACKAGING AND DISPENSING OF SUPPLIES

42. If a muslin-wrapped item is sterilized and then sealed in an airtight plastic bag, the shelf life

A. remains at 14–21 days
B. remains at 21–30 days
C. can be prolonged for 3–6 months
D. can be prolonged for 6–12 months

43. Which of the following is *not* an acceptable wrapper for gas sterilization?

A. nylon
B. muslin
C. paper
D. plastic

44. All of the following are acceptable methods of sealing a package for sterilization *except*

A. heat sealing
B. pressure-sensitive tape
C. peel-open seal
D. staples

45. Which of the following is the only acceptable plastic that can be used for a steam sterilization wrapper?

A. polyethylene
B. polypropylene
C. polyamide
D. polyvinyl chloride

46. Which of the following statements regarding a nonwoven fabric wrapper is true?

A. it is expensive because it is a one-use item
B. it needs frequent inspection and repair
C. it provides no barrier against moisture
D. it has memory

47. Which of the following statements regarding muslin wrappers is false?

A. muslin must be laundered, even if unused, in order to rehydrate it
B. a 140-thread count of unbleached muslin is used for wrappers
C. muslin is flexible and easy to handle
D. small holes can be repaired by stitching on a patch

48. Packages wrapped in muslin must have

A. one layer
B. two layers
C. three layers
D. four layers

49. The maximum storage life for a muslin-wrapped item in a closed cabinet is

A. 7 days
B. 14 days
C. 21 days
D. 30 days

50. All of the following are true of paper wrappers *except* that they

A. provide a good long-term barrier
B. are disposable
C. are inexpensive
D. are easy to open and handle

51. The best means of determining effective steam sterilizer function is

A. biologic monitoring
B. paper indicators
C. graph of the sterilizing cycle
D. pressure-sensitive tape

52. When using a pour solution

A. a portion may be poured and the cap replaced
B. the contents must be used or discarded after the bottle is opened
C. the cap may be replaced if it has not been placed on an unsterile surface
D. the solution may be used on the same case as long as the cap is not replaced

53. What is the standard safety margin on package wrappers?

A. up to the edge
B. less than 1 inch
C. 1 inch or more
D. none of the above

54. Which is *not* considered an acceptable technique when using a peel-packaged item?

A. the ends of the flaps are secured in the hand of the circulator so they do not dangle
B. the wrapper may be pulled back, not torn, to expose the sterile contents
C. the sterile person may lift the contents out of the package by reaching down and lifting straight up
D. the circulator may slide the item across the wrapper edge onto the sterile field

55. When opening a wrapper, the circulator should open the

A. corner nearest the body first
B. corner farthest from the body first
C. corner farthest from the body last
D. sides of the package first

56. When the scrub nurse opens an inner sterile wrapper

A. the side nearest the body is opened first
B. the side nearest the body is opened last
C. the lateral areas are done first
D. A or B

57. When flipping a sterile item onto a sterile field, the circulator may

A. lean over the field if the package is difficult to handle
B. never reach over the sterile field and shake the item out
C. reach over a basin set to shake the item out
D. lean over the linen pack to shake the item out

C. ENVIRONMENTAL CONTROL

58. A glass suction bottle should ideally be

A. rinsed with tap water between each case
B. cleaned with a disinfectant solution and autoclaved before reuse
C. rinsed with sterile distilled water between each case
D. autoclaved daily

59. Excessive exposure to radiation can affect the

A. skin
B. brain
C. ovaries
D. stomach

60. Open shelving must be cleaned with a germicide

A. each case
B. each day
C. each week
D. each month

61. While a surgical case is in progress

A. doors remain open so staff can easily move in or out
B. doors should remain closed
C. doors remain open to circulate air
D. doors may be opened or closed

62. An agent widely used for OR housekeeping is a/an

A. chlorine compound solution
B. formaldehyde solution
C. glutaraldehyde solution
D. iodophor solution

63. The room temperature in an OR should be

A. below 50°F
B. below 60°F
C. between 68 and 80°F
D. between 80 and 86°F

64. When cleaning the floor between cases

A. a clean mop head must be used each time
B. a two-bucket system, one detergent and one clear water, is used
C. buckets must be emptied and cleaned between case
D. all of the above

65. If an OR staff member wears eyeglasses

A. the glasses should be wiped with an antiseptic solution before each operation
B. the glasses should be soaked for 5 minutes in an antiseptic solution before the day begins
C. the glasses should be wiped with an antiseptic solution daily
D. no special care is necessary

66. If a lab coat is worn when an OR staff member leaves the OR suite,

A. it must be clean, closed, and knee-length
B. the underneath OR attire must be changed upon re-entry to the OR
C. the underneath OR attire does not need to be changed upon re-entry to the OR
D. A and B

67. The most effective OR attire is

A. a loose-fitting dress
B. a snug-fitting dress
C. trousers with tight-fitting cuffs
D. trousers with loose-fitting cuffs

68. The most effective protection from the radiation of x-rays is

A. lead apron
B. double thick muslin apron
C. 3-foot distance from machine
D. 3-foot distance from patient

69. It is considered good technique to

A. change the mask only if it becomes moistened
B. hang the mask around the neck
C. criss-cross the strings over the head
D. handle the mask only by the strings

70. Jewelry should be prohibited in the OR because

A. it can scratch a patient
B. it can catch on OR equipment
C. it is a reservoir for bacteria
D. all of the above

71. A surgical hat is put on

A. before the OR suit or dress
B. after the OR suit or dress
C. when the OR suite is entered
D. before leaving the OR area

72. Sterile gloves

A. should be wiped off after donning to remove lubricant
B. need not be wiped off
C. should be wiped off only in septic cases
D. should be wiped off only in eye cases

73. Electrical cords should be

A. removed from outlets by the cord
B. wrapped tightly around equipment
C. removed from pathways so equipment is not rolled over them
D. disconnected from the unit before disconnection from the wall

74. Combustible anesthetic gases may be administered in the presence of

A. cautery
B. endothermy
C. radiographic equipment
D. air-powered equipment

75. Each of the following would need to be present for an explosion to occur *except*

A. oxygen
B. a source of ignition
C. carbon dioxide
D. a flammable gas, vapor, or liquid

76. Which of the following creates a potential explosion hazard in the OR when a flammable anesthetic is used?

A. friction of drapes on the reservoir bag of the anesthesia machine
B. cotton blankets and clothing
C. motion around the anesthesia equipment and the patient's head
D. A and C

77. The first action that must be taken in the event a fire occurs in a room during surgery is to

A. evacuate the patient and personnel
B. move the burning article from proximity to the oxygen source and anesthesia machine
C. bring in a fire extinguisher
D. pull the fire alarm

78. The result attained by touching a grounded person during a surgical procedure that involves a flammable anesthetic agent is to

A. provide conductivity
B. ground the staff member
C. ground the patient
D. dissipate static charge

D. ASEPTIC TECHNIQUE IN GENERAL PROCEDURES

79. The minimum distance which a nonsterile person should remain from a sterile field is

A. 6 inches
B. 1 foot
C. 2 feet
D. 3 feet

80. Transfer forceps are

A. not considered safe to use routinely
B. safe to use
C. safe to use if solution is changed daily
D. recommended for removal of instruments from the flash autoclave

81. Tables are considered sterile

A. on the top and 2 inches below the table level
B. up to 2 feet off the ground
C. on the top and in the area that has been pulled close to the sterile field
D. only on the top

82. Gowns are considered sterile only from

A. waist to neck level in front, and back, and the sleeves
B. waist to shoulder, front and back, and the sleeves
C. neck to thighs in front, and the sleeves
D. waist to shoulder level in front, and the sleeves

83. Suction tubing is attached to the drapes with a/an

A. towel clip
B. nonperforating clamp
C. Kocher clamp
D. Allis clamp

84. At the end of the case, drapes should be

A. pulled off and placed in a hamper
B. rolled off and placed on the floor so they can be checked for instruments
C. rolled off and placed in a hamper
D. checked for instruments, rolled off, and placed in a hamper

85. During surgery, towel clips

A. may be removed only by the circulator
B. may not be removed once fastened
C. may be removed and discarded as long as the area is covered with sterile linen
D. may be removed and discarded from the field

86. As grossly soiled instruments are returned to the scrub, they should be

A. placed in a basin of sterile saline to soak off debris
B. wiped off with a moist sponge or soaked in a basin of sterile distilled water
C. wiped off with a dry sponge
D. discarded so that the circulator can clean them thoroughly

87. Which of the following actions by the scrub nurse is *not* an acceptable sterile technique principle?

A. discard tubing that falls below sterile field edges without touching the contaminated part
B. reach behind sterile team members to retrieve instruments so they do not collect on the patient
C. face sterile areas when passing them
D. step away from the sterile field if contaminated

88. When the scrub is draping a nonsterile table, he or she must

A. cover the back edge of the table first
B. use a single-thickness drape
C. be sure the drape touches the floor
D. cuff the drape over his or her gloved hands

89. When covering a Mayo stand, the scrub should

A. use a wide cuff
B. use no cuff
C. open the cover fully before placement
D. ask the circulator to pull on the cover

90. If a sterile field becomes moistened during a case

A. nothing can be done
B. extra linen is added to area
C. the wet sections are removed and replaced with dry
D. the wet sections are covered with a plastic adherent drape

91. Which statement regarding a grounding plate for electrosurgery is false?

A. the plate must have good contact with the patient's skin
B. the plate must be lubricated with electrosurgical gel
C. the plate must be placed directly over a bony prominence
D. the grounded pathway returns the electrical current to the unit after the surgeon delivers it to the operative site

92. Nosocomial infection refers to

A. infections generating from the nose
B. hospital-acquired infections
C. home-acquired infections
D. invasion of microbes capable of causing disease

93. When a sterile item is hanging or extending over the sterile table edge, the scrub nurse

A. must watch closely that no one comes near it
B. does not touch the part hanging below table level
C. should pull it back onto the table so it does not become contaminated
D. may use the item

94. If a sterile package falls to the floor

A. it may be used if the floor is clean and dry
B. it may be used if the wrapper is linen
C. it must be discarded
D. it may be used if the wrapper is paper or plastic

95. Which of the following is considered a break in technique?

A. a sterile person turns his back to a nonsterile person or area when passing
B. sterile persons face sterile areas
C. a sterile person sits or leans against a nonsterile surface
D. nonsterile persons avoid sterile areas

96. In which situation would sterility be questionable?

    A. if a sterilized pack is found in an unsterile workroom
    B. if the surgeon turns away from the sterile field for a brow wipe
    C. if the scrub drapes a nonsterile table, covering the edge nearest the body first
    D. if the lip of a pour bottle is held over the basin as close to the edge as possible

97. Which statement regarding sterile technique is true?

    A. sterile persons may lean on sterile tables or the draped person
    B. unsterile persons pass the sterile field with back towards it
    C. only the surface level of table covers are sterile
    D. a sterile person passes a sterile area with back towards it

98. Which condition regarding sterile technique is *not* recommended?

    A. sterile tables are set up just prior to the operation
    B. sterile tables may be set up and safely covered until time of surgery
    C. once sterile packs are open, someone must remain in the room to maintain vigilance
    D. sterile persons pass each other back to back

99. Which of the following conditions is *not* an acceptable aseptic technique?

    A. scrub nurse standing on a platform or standing stool
    B. scrub nurse keeps hands below shoulder level
    C. scrub nurse folds arms with hands at axillae
    D. scrub nurse's hands are at or above waist level

100. If the surgeon sutures on the skin towels, the scrub nurse should

    A. discard the needle and holder from the field
    B. wrap the needle and holder in a towel and place next to the skin knife
    C. pass the needle from the field
    D. follow no special procedure

101. When handing drapes to the surgeon, where should the scrub stand in relation to the surgeon?

    A. on the opposite side of the table
    B. on the same side of the table
    C. at the foot of the table
    D. any position is acceptable

102. The Mayo stand should

    A. remain sterile until the patient leaves the room

    B. be pulled away from the sterile field by the circulator after skin closure
    C. be completely emptied immediately after skin closure
    D. be considered unsterile once the dressing is applied

103. Which statement regarding drying the hands and arms after a surgical scrub is false?

    A. bend forward, holding hands and elbows above the waist
    B. open the towel full length
    C. dry in a rotating motion
    D. dry thoroughly, doing cleanest area last

104. Which statement is false regarding gowning another person?

    A. open the hand towel and lay it on the person's hand
    B. hand the folded gown to the person at the neckband
    C. keep hands on the outside of the gown under a protective cuff
    D. release the gown once the person touches it

105. The scrub procedure fulfills all of the following conditions *except*

    A. reduces the microbial count
    B. leaves an antimicrobial residue
    C. renders the skin aseptic
    D. removes skin oil

106. If the scrub nurse needs to change a glove during an operation

    A. the scrub must not turn away from the sterile field
    B. the circulator pulls the glove off
    C. the scrub pulls the glove off
    D. the scrub uses closed-glove technique to reapply gloves

107. Which statement regarding the removal of gown and gloves is false?

    A. the gloves are removed before the gown
    B. the gown is pulled off inside-out
    C. the gown is untied by the circulator
    D. gloves are removed inside-out

108. Which surgical scrub method is considered the most effective?

    A. time method
    B. brush-stroke method
    C. 3-minute anatomic method
    D. A and B

109. Which of the following statements regarding preparation for a surgical scrub is false?

  A. fingernails should not reach beyond fingertip
  B. nail polish may be worn if freshly applied
  C. anyone with a cut, abrasion, or hangnail should not scrub
  D. a nonoil-base hand lotion may be used to protect the skin

110. Nail cleaners

  A. should be metal or disposable plastic
  B. should be orangewood sticks
  C. must be sterilized between uses
  D. A and C

111. When carrying out the scrub procedure, all of the following are true *except*

  A. hands are held above the levels of the elbows
  B. small amounts of water are added during the scrub to develop suds and remove detritus
  C. the arm is scrubbed in a back-and-forth motion
  D. all steps of the scrub procedure begin with the hands and end with the elbows

112. The surgical scrub is

  A. sterilization of the skin
  B. mechanical cleansing of the skin
  C. chemical cleansing of the skin
  D. mechanical washing and chemical antisepsis of the skin

113. Scrub technique ends

  A. 2 inches below the elbow
  B. just below the elbow
  C. at the elbow
  D. 2 inches above the elbow

114. Which statement regarding sterility is false?

  A. wrapper edges are unsterile
  B. instruments or sutures hanging over the table edge are discarded
  C. sterile persons pass each other back to back
  D. a sterile person faces a nonsterile person when passing

115. Which of the following is *not* acceptable technique in draping?

  A. hold the drapes high until directly over the proper area
  B. protect the gloved hands by cuffing the end of the drape over them
  C. unfold the drapes before bringing them to the OR table
  D. place the drapes on a dry area

116. When draping a table, the scrub nurse should drape

  A. back to front
  B. front to back
  C. side to side
  D. either A or B

117. When handing the skin towels to the surgeon, the scrub should

  A. stand on the opposite side of the table from the surgeon
  B. stand at the foot of the table
  C. stand on the same side of the table as the surgeon
  D. stand toward the head of the table

118. If a drape is placed incorrectly it

  A. is discarded by the scrub
  B. is peeled off by the circulator
  C. is covered over with another drape
  D. may be adjusted correctly

119. Draping is always done from _____ to _____, draping _____ first.

  A. an unsterile area, a sterile area, nearest
  B. an unsterile area, a sterile area, farthest
  C. a sterile area, an unsterile area, farthest
  D. a sterile area, an unsterile area, nearest

120. The skin prep for a breast biopsy is

  A. routine
  B. done gently
  C. done vigorously
  D. eliminated

121. Cancer technique in surgery refers to

  A. the administration of an anticancer drug directly into the cancer site
  B. the discarding of instruments coming in contact with tumor after each use
  C. the use of radiation therapy at the time of surgery
  D. the identification of the lesion

122. If an x-ray cassette is used within the sterile field it must be

  A. encased in a sterile cover
  B. sterilized in the flash autoclave
  C. cold sterilized
  D. wrapped in sterile gauze

123. Which item is removed first following a surgical procedure?

A. gown
B. gloves
C. mask
D. booties

124. A common radiopaque contrast medium used in the OR is

A. barium sulfate
B. Ritalin
C. Baralyme
D. Renografin

125. A postoperative complication attributed to glove powder entering a wound is

A. granulomata
B. infection
C. inflammation
D. keloid formation

126. Which of the following is *not* an adequate method of protection of OR personnel from radiation exposure?

A. line the walls of rooms and fixed equipment with lead
B. personnel should stand 3 feet or more from the patient and out of the direct beam during exposure
C. sterile team members stand behind a lead screen, nonsterile team leaves the room
D. lead-lined aprons should be worn

127. Each of the following would require two setups *except*

A. breast biopsy and radical
B. abdominoperineal resection
C. D & C and laparotomy
D. vein ligation and stripping

128. Which statement is false regarding the preparation of the patient for a skin graft?

A. the recipient site is scrubbed first
B. the donor site is prepared with a colorless antiseptic agent
C. separate setups are necessary for skin preparation of recipient and donor sites
D. items used in preparation of the recipient site must not be permitted to contaminate the donor site

129. When drop technique for an intestinal procedure is utilized

A. two Mayo stands are used

B. drapes and gloves do not need to be changed
C. contaminated instruments are discarded, gloves are changed, and the incisional area is redraped
D. a separate setup is used for the closure

130. Which of the following methods of intestinal technique provides the greatest margin of safety?

A. drop technique method
B. clean-closure method
C. redrape method
D. regowning and gloving method

131. Ideally, operating room floors should be flooded with _____ and _____ at the end of each case.

A. detergent-disinfectant, wet-vacuumed
B. germicidal solution, mopped
C. germicidal solution, wet-vaccumed
D. detergent-disinfectant, mopped

132. When a case is completed

A. only soiled linen is discarded into the linen hamper
B. all linen is discarded into the linen hamper
C. wet linen is placed in the center of the linen bundle
D. B and C

133. Between cases, nondisposable suction bottles should be

A. emptied and washed before reuse
B. emptied, decontaminated, washed, and autoclaved before reuse
C. emptied if more than half full
D. emptied before reuse

134. If terminal sterilization facilities are not in a room immediately adjacent to the OR suite, the procedure for transporting soiled instruments is

A. scrub removes gown, covers instruments with a clean towel or sheet, and transports them to cleaning area
B. scrub keeps gown on and transports instruments to cleaning area
C. scrub keeps gown on, covers instruments with a clean towel or sheet, and transports instruments to cleaning area
D. scrub washes instruments in OR suite and then transports them to terminal sterilization area

Answers and Explanations

A. STERILIZATION, DISINFECTION, AND ANTISEPSIS

1. **(A)** Fifteen pounds of pressure is necessary in the steam sterilizer set at 250°F. It is 27 psi if it were set at 270°F. *(11:37)*

2. **(B)** In gravity displacement, steam enters the autoclave under pressure at the rear of the sterilizer, forcing the heavier air ahead of it down and forward until it is discharged from a port at the front of the sterilizer. *(25:42)*

3. **(A)** Positive assurance that sterile conditions have been achieved by either steam, ethylene oxide, or dry heat sterilization can be obtained only through a biologic control test. These should be done at least weekly. The most dependable is a preparation of living spores resistant to the sterilizing agent. *(2:105)*

4. **(C)** After the door is opened, the load is left untouched to dry for 10 to 30 minutes. Warm packages laid on a solid, cold surface become damp from steam condensation and thus are contaminated. The time required depends on the type and size of load. *(2:100)*

5. **(C)** Instruments wrapped as a set in double-thickness wrappers are autoclaved at a setting of 250°F for 30 minutes. It would be 15 minutes at a 270°F setting. *(2:99)*

6. **(B)** In a flash (high-speed pressure) sterilizer set at 270°F, the minimum exposure time is 3 minutes for unwrapped items. With this cycle, the entire time for starting, sterilizing, etc., is 6 to 7 minutes. *(2:94)*

7. **(D)** Rubber tubing should not be folded or kinked because steam cannot penetrate it nor displace air from folds. A residual of distilled water should be left in the lumen. Rubber bands must not be used around solid items as steam cannot penetrate through or under rubber. *(2:95-96)*

8. **(A)** Linen packs must not weigh more than 12 pounds. Linen must be freshly laundered. Items must be fan-folded or loosely rolled. *(2:95)*

9. **(B)** Steam sterilization is the easiest, safest, surest, and fastest method of sterilization. No item should be gassed that can be steamed. *(2:93-95)*

10. **(D)** The high-vacuum sterilizer temperatures are controlled at 272 to 276°F. Air is evacuated by a pump and a steam ejector system which helps eliminate air from the package. *(2:94)*

11. **(A)** The washer-sterilizer washes and terminally sterilizes items immediately after an operation is completed. Steam under pressure floods the chamber to sterilize the items at 270°F. It can also be used just as a flash sterilizer. *(2:94)*

12. **(B)** The ultrasonic cleaner (which is not a sterilizer) utilizes ultrasonic energy and high-frequency sound waves. Instruments are cleaned by cavitation. In this process tiny bubbles are generated by high-frequency sound waves. Instruments are cleaned by cavitation. In this process tiny bubbles are generated by high-frequency sound waves. These bubbles generate minute vacuum areas that dislodge, dissolve, or disperse soil. *(2:95)*

13. **(C)** Hinged instruments must be open with box locks unlocked to permit steam contact on all surfaces. All detachable parts should be disassembled. *(2:95)*

14. **(D)** Solutions are sterilized alone on a slow exhaust cycle to prevent them from boiling over. The pressure gauge must read 0°F before opening the door. This is so the caps will not pop off. *(2:99)*

15. **(D)** Wrapped basin sets are sterilized at 250°F for a minimum of 20 minutes. They are placed on their sides to allow air flow out of them. This also helps water flow out. *(2:99)*

16. **(A)** Basins and solid utensils must be separated by a porous material if they are nested, to permit permeation of steam around all surfaces, and condensation of steam from the inside during sterilization. Sponges or linen are not packaged in basins. *(2:95)*

17. **(B)** EO gas is an effective substitute for most items that cannot be sterilized by heat or that would be damaged by repeated exposure to heat. It is noncorrosive and does not damage items. It completely penetrates porous materials. *(2:100–101)*

18. **(D)** Dry heat (hot air) is used primarily to sterilize anhydrous oils, petroleum products, and bulk powders that steam and gas cannot penetrate. Microbial death is caused by a physical oxidation or slow burning up process by coagulation of the protein in the cells. *(2:104)*

19. **(D)** Ethylene oxide gas is used to sterilize items that are either heat or moisture sensitive. It is colorless and has an odor similar to ether. It has an inhalation toxicity. *(2:100; 32:58)*

20. **(D)** A major disadvantage of ETO is the long aeration time required on absorbent materials. These include such items as rubber, plastic, polyethylene, or silicone. It is a complicated process and should only be used if other methods are inappropriate. *(2:101)*

21. **(C)** Nonporous items of metals and glass may be used immediately and do not require aeration. Rubber requires aeration. The length of time is dependent on the thickness of the item and its intended use as well. *(2:103)*

22. **(A)** Some products that are commercially available are sterilized by irradiation (ionizing radiation). Ionic energy is produced which converts to thermal and chemical energy. This has a lethal effect on microorganisms. *(2:105)*

23. **(A)** EO gas is highly flammable and explosive in air. By diluting it with an inert gas such as a fluorinated hydrocarbon or carbon dioxide, a safe, nonflammable agent is provided. *(2:100)*

24. **(A)** Formaldehyde is sporicidal in a minimum of 12 hours, whereas the iodophors, alcohols, and phenols do not have this quality. *(2:108–110)*

25. **(D)** Cobalt 60 is a radioactive isotope which produces gamma rays. It is the most commonly used source for irradiation sterilization. The gamma rays are electromagnetic waves. *(2:105)*

26. **(C)** Gas sterilizers usually operate at 120 to 140°F. Temperature influences the destruction of microorganisms. As temperature is increased, exposure time can be decreased; however, 140°F is the uppermost temperature limit for many heat-sensitive materials. *(2:100)*

27. **(A)** Items must be thoroughly rinsed before use. Solution is reusable for the time set by the manufacturer. Items must be clean and dry before submersion. *(2:103–104)*

28. **(B)** Aqueous Cidex is an activated glutaraldehyde solution; it is used as a choice method for sterilizing heat-sensitive items that cannot be sterilized by steam or if an EO gas sterilizer is not available. It is a high level disinfectant. *(2:103; 32:64)*

29. **(A)** Mercurial compounds and quaternary ammonium compounds are not recommended for hospital use because the hazards outweigh their effectiveness in the hospital environment. *(2:110)*

30. **(D)** Alcohol does not leave a residue on treated surfaces. It is bactericidal, pseudomonicidal, and fungicidal in a minimum of 10 minutes' exposure and is tuberculocidal and virucidal for all viruses in a minimum of 15 minutes' exposure. It can never be used on lensed instruments with cement mountings because it dissolves the cement. *(2:108)*

31. **(D)** Endogenic means having origin within a cell or organism. It concerns spore forming within the bacterial cell. *(36:545)*

32. **(C)** Staphene or O-Syl are phenolic detergents. Phenol is carbolic acid. As a disinfectant, it is effective even in the presence of organic matter such as blood, feces, and tissue debris. *(17:36–37)*

33. **(C)** Immersion in a 2% aqueous solution of activated, buffered alkaline glutaraldehyde is sporicidal (kills spores) within 10 hours. It is chosen for heat-sensitive items that cannot be steamed or if ETO is unavailable or impractical. *(2:103)*

34. **(C)** Activated glutaraldehyde solution is bactericidal, pseudomonicidal, tuberculocidal, fungicidal, and virucidal in 10 minutes for disinfection. It is sporicidal within 10 hours. Ten hours is required for sterilization. *(2:103–104)*

35. **(B)** Lumens of instruments or tubing must be completely filled with solution. All items should be placed in a container deep enough to completely immerse them. All items should be dry before immersion so that the solution is not diluted. *(2:104)*

36. **(C)** Moisture is essential in gas sterilization. Desiccated or highly dried bacterial spores are resistant to EO gas; therefore, they must be hydrated in order for the gas to be effective.   *(2:100)*

37. **(C)** The size of the chamber and the contents will determine the exposure period in a gravity displacement sterilizer; however, the minimum is 15 minutes. Most autoclaves operate on a standard cycle of 250 to 254°F. The psis are 15 to 17 pounds.   *(2:94)*

38. **(B)** Chemical indicators or sterilization indicators do not prove sterility but can be utilized to detect an improperly functioning autoclave. The tape changes color when exposed to the sterilization agent for a certain time and temperature; however, this only identifies packages that have been exposed to the physical conditions of a sterilization cycle. A more accurate method such as biologic control is necessary to check sterilizer effectiveness.   *(32:56)*

39. **(B)** Aeration following EO sterilization can be accomplished at room temperature; however, aeration of exposed items at an elevated temperature (in an aerator) enhances the dissipation rate of absorbed gases, resulting in faster removal. The aerator is a separate unit.   *(2:101–103)*

40. **(A)** EO or ETO is a chemical agent that kills microorganisms, including spores. It interferes with the normal metabolism of protein and reproductive processes, resulting in cell death.   *(2:100)*

41. **(C)** Items must be clean and free from grease and oil to be effective. This is a disadvantage especially on items that need greasing or oiling to function properly.   *(2:93)*

B. PACKAGING AND DISPENSING OF SUPPLIES

42. **(D)** Muslin-wrapped items may be stored from 21 to 30 days, then resterilization is required. However, if these items are sealed in an airtight plastic bag immediately after sterilization (following cooling and aerating), their shelf-life can be prolonged from 6 to 12 months. This cover may not have cracks or holes.   *(2:106)*

43. **(A)** Nylon is not used for EO sterilization because of inadequate permeability; however, muslin, nonwoven fabric, paper, and plastic are safely used. Items wrapped for gas sterilization should be tagged to avoid inadvertent steam sterilization.   *(2:102)*

44. **(D)** Staples, pins, paper clips, or other penetrating objects must never be used to seal packages. They cannot be removed without destroying package integrity. Contamination of contents would occur.   *(2:96)*

45. **(B)** Polypropylene film of 1 to 3 mm thickness is the only plastic acceptable for steam sterilization. It is used in the form of pouches presealed on two or three sides. The open sides are then heat-sealed.   *(2:98)*

46. **(A)** Nonwoven fabric wrappers are disposable, eliminating the need for inspection and repair. They provide an excellent barrier against microorganisms and moisture. They are expensive because they are one-use items, but easy to handle with very little memory.   *(2:97)*

47. **(D)** Small holes can be heat-sealed with double-vulcanized patches; they never can be stitched because this will leave needle holes in the muslin.   *(2:97)*

48. **(D)** Muslin wrappers must have two layers of double thickness (four thicknesses) to serve as a sufficient dust filter and microbial barrier. A 140-thread count unbleached muslin is used for wrappers. They are sewn together at edges.   *(2:97)*

49. **(D)** The storage life for muslin is 30 days maximum in closed cabinets. Muslin wets easily and dries quickly so water stains may not be obvious.   *(2:97)*

50. **(D)** Paper wrappers are disposable, inexpensive, and provide a good long-term barrier. However, it is difficult to spread them open so that contents can be removed easily and safely. They have memory and flip back easily. They are easy to puncture or tear.   *(2:98)*

51. **(A)** Biologic monitoring is the best means of determining effective sterilizer functioning. Because they take time to do, they cannot be the only control method.   *(11:54–55)*

52. **(B)** After a sterile bottle is opened, the contents must be used or discarded. The cap cannot be replaced without contamination of pouring edges. The edges of anything that encloses sterile contents are considered unsterile.   *(2:88)*

53. **(C)** A 1-inch safety margin is usually considered standard on package wrappers. After a package is open, the edges are unsterile.   *(32:48)*

54. **(D)** Contents of peel packs should be flipped or lifted upward and never permitted to slide over the edges. The inner edge of the heat seal is considered the line of demarcation between sterile and unsterile. Flaps on peel-open packages should be pulled back, not torn.   *(2:88)*

55. **(B)** A sterile article is opened by the circulating nurse by opening the corner farthest from the body first, and the corner nearest the body last.   *(32:48)*

56. **(A)** When a scrub nurse opens a sterile wrapper, the side nearest the body is opened first. The portion of the drape then protects the gown, enabling the nurse to move closer to the table to open the opposite side. *(32:48)*

57. **(B)** When flipping a sterile item onto a sterile field, the circulator may never reach over the sterile field and shake the item from the package. *(2:143)*

C. ENVIRONMENTAL CONTROL

58. **(B)** Glass suction bottles should be thoroughly cleaned with a disinfectant solution and autoclaved before reuse; however, if the supply does not allow for a sterilized bottle for each procedure, they should be thoroughly washed with a disinfectant solution between rinses and terminally sterilized at the end of the day. *(11:10)*

59. **(C)** Excessive exposure to radiation can affect active blood-forming organs, gonads, and the ocular lens. *(36:1448)*

60. **(B)** Open shelving should be cleaned and wiped with a germicide daily. *(11:9)*

61. **(B)** Doors should be closed during and in between cases to reduce the microbial count. *(2:115)*

62. **(D)** Iodophors are used in housekeeping, as disinfectants for floors, and other inanimate objects. *(2:101)*

63. **(C)** Room temperature is maintained within a range of 68 to 80°F. *(2:115)*

64. **(D)** A wet vacuum system is the best. However, if mopping is to be utilized, a clean mop is used. Each time the mop is used, a two-bucket system is recommended (one a detergent-germicide and the other clear water), and the buckets must be emptied and cleaned between uses. *(11:9)*

65. **(A)** Eyeglasses should be cleaned with an antiseptic solution before each operation to prevent cross-contamination. *(2:122)*

66. **(D)** A lab coat may be worn over the OR suit when leaving the OR. However, it must be clean and not hung in a locker with street clothes. It also must be kept buttoned. The suit must be changed upon return to the suite. *(2:122)*

67. **(C)** Trousers with tight-fitting cuffs at the ankles are considered the best barrier against bacterial shedding from the perineum. If dresses are worn, the women must wear panty hose. *(11:11)*

68. **(A)** Lead-lined aprons should be worn to protect the staff from radiation especially during the use of image intensifier. Thyroid collars are also particularly useful for protection. *(2:296)*

69. **(D)** Masks should be handled only by the strings, thereby keeping the facial area of the mask clean. The mask should never be worn around the neck. Upper strings are tied at the top of the head; lower strings are tied behind the neck because criss-crossing distorts mask contours and makes the mask less efficient. *(2:123)*

70. **(D)** Jewelry is dangerous because it can scratch a patient, catch on equipment, and is a reservoir for bacteria. An added hazard is that exposed dangle-type necklaces, earrings, or bracelets could fall onto a sterile field. *(11:13)*

71. **(A)** A cap or hood is put on before a scrub suit or dress in order to protect the garment from contamination by hair. *(2:123)*

72. **(A)** Gloves are prelubricated with an absorbable dry powder before sterilization. This lubricant may at times cause serious complications (such as granulomas or peritonitis) if it is introduced to wounds. Therefore, gloves should be thoroughly wiped with a sterile damp towel or terry washcloth after donning. *(2:124)*

73. **(C)** Electrical cords should not be kinked, curled, or tightly wrapped. They should be handled by the plug, not the cord, when disconnecting. Always remove cords from pathways before rolling in equipment as this can break the cord. *(32:31)*

74. **(D)** Combustible anesthetics should not be administered in the presence of cautery, endothermy, or radiographic equipment. *(32:32)*

75. **(C)** An explosion is a result of the combination of oxygen, a source of ignition, and a flammable gas, vapor, or liquid. *(2:286)*

76. **(D)** In order to reduce the explosion hazard, all unnecessary motion in the area around the anesthesia equipment and the patient's head should be avoided. Avoid friction on the reservoir bag of the anesthesia machine and see that drapes do not touch the bag or cover the machine. *(2:287)*

77. **(B)** Should fire occur in a room during an operation, the burning article must be removed immediately from proximity to the oxygen or anesthetic sources to prevent explosion. *(2:116)*

78. **(D)** In order to dissipate static charge when a flammable anesthetic is used, anyone who must make contact with either the patient or the anesthesiologist does so by first touching the anesthesiologist's back or stool, the operating table, or the patient at least 2 feet from the face mask. *(2:287)*

D. ASEPTIC TECHNIQUE IN GENERAL PROCEDURES

79. **(B)** All unsterile persons should remain at least 1 foot from any sterile surface. *(2:148)*

80. **(A)** The routine use of transfer forceps is considered obsolete. They may be used if they are wrapped separately and discarded after each use. *(2:143)*

81. **(D)** A sterile draped table is considered sterile only on the top. The edges and sides extending below table level are considered unsterile. *(2:87)*

82. **(D)** Gowns are considered sterile only from the waist to shoulder level in front, and the sleeves. *(2:87)*

83. **(B)** Suction tubing is attached to the drapes with a nonperforating clamp. *(2:140)*

84. **(D)** Check drapes for instruments. Roll drapes off the patient to prevent sparking and airborne contamination. Wet areas should be placed in the center to prevent soaking through the laundry bag. *(2:154)*

85. **(C)** Once a clip has been fastened through a drape, do not remove it because the points are contaminated. If it is necessary to remove one during a case, discard it from the field and cover the area with a piece of sterile linen. *(2:140)*

86. **(B)** Old blood and debris should be removed from instruments as soon as possible with water so that it does not dry on surfaces or crevices. *(2:280)*

87. **(B)** Scrub persons should not reach behind a member of the sterile team. They may go around the person, passing back to back. *(2:141)*

88. **(D)** In draping a nonsterile table, the scrub nurse should cuff the drape over her gloved hand in preparation for opening it. The side of the drape towards her is done first to minimize the possibility of contaminating the front of the gown. *(2:136)*

89. **(A)** A wide cuff is used on the Mayo cover to protect the gloved hands. *(2:136)*

90. **(B)** The table and sterile field should be kept as dry as possible. However, extra towels may be spread if a solution has soaked through a sterile drape. *(2:90, 141)*

91. **(C)** The ground plate or inactive electrode is lubricated with an electrosurgical gel and is placed in good contact with a fleshy, nonhairy body surface. It should not be placed over a bony prominence. The grounded pathway returns the electrical current to the unit after the surgeon delivers it to the operative site. *(2:34)*

92. **(B)** Nosocomial infections are infections that patients acquire during hospitalization. *(2:75)*

93. **(B)** Anything falling or extending over a table edge is unsterile. The scrub person does not touch the part hanging below table level. *(2:87)*

94. **(C)** If a sterile package falls to the floor, it must be discarded because its sterility is doubtful. *(2:87)*

95. **(C)** Sitting or leaning against a nonsterile surface is a break in technique since a sterile person should keep contact with nonsterile areas to a minimum. *(2:89)*

96. **(A)** If sterility is doubtful, consider it not sterile. Do not use a pack, even if it appears to be sterile, if it is found in a nonsterile workroom. *(2:87)*

97. **(C)** Only the top of a sterile draped table is considered sterile. *(2:87)*

98. **(B)** Covering sterile tables for later use is not recommended because it is difficult to uncover a table without contamination. *(2:89)*

99. **(C)** Hands are kept at or above waist level, away from the face and arms, and never folded, because there may be perspiration in the axillary region. *(2:87)*

100. **(A)** When a surgeon sutures the skin towels in place, the needle and needleholder are discarded from the sterile field. *(2:139)*

101. **(B)** The scrub who hands the drapes to the surgeon should stand on the same side of the table in order to avoid reaching over the unsterile OR table. *(2:136, 139)*

102. **(A)** The Mayo stand and instrument table are pushed away from the OR table as soon as the intermediate layer of the dressing is applied. The Mayo stand should not be contaminated until the patient has left the room. A knife handle, tissue forceps, scissors, four hemostats, and two Allis forceps should remain on the Mayo in the event that the patient has a cardiac arrest, hemorrhage, or other emergency in the immediate postoperative period. *(2:141, 142, 153)*

103. **(D)** Dry both hands thoroughly but independently. Dry each arm using a rotating motion while moving up the arm to the elbow; do not retrace the area. Bend forward slightly from the waist, holding hands and elbows above the waist and away from the body. The towel should be opened full length and reversed for each arm. *(2:128)*

104. **(B)** Before handling a gown, unfold it carefully, holding it at the neckband. *(2:132)*

105. **(C)** The surgical scrub removes skin oil, reduces the microbial count, and leaves an antimicrobial residue on the skin. The skin can never be rendered sterile (aseptic); it is considered surgically clean. *(32:73)*

106. **(B)** To change a glove during an operation the scrub nurse must turn away from the sterile field. The circulator pulls the glove off inside-out, and open-glove technique is used to don a new pair of gloves *(2:133)*

107. **(A)** The gown is always removed before the gloves. It is pulled downward from the shoulders, turning the sleeves inside out as it is pulled off the arms, gloves are turned inside out, using glove-to-glove then skin-to-skin technique as they are removed. The circulating nurse unfastens the neck and waist. *(2:133)*

108. **(D)** Either the time method or brush-stroke method is effective if properly executed. If hospital policy dictates a 10-minute initial scrub, the 5-minute scrub may be used for subsequent operations. However, studies have shown that a vigorous 5-minute scrub with a reliable agent is as effective as the 10-minute scrub. *(2:126–127)*

109. **(B)** Chipped nail polish harbors microorganisms. No polish is preferred. *(2:126)*

110. **(D)** Nail cleaners should be metal or plastic single-use disposable. Reusable nail cleaners must be sterilized between uses. Orangewood sticks should not be used because the wood may splinter and harbor *Pseudomonas*. Also wood does not sterilize properly. *(2:125)*

111. **(C)** The arm is scrubbed using a circular motion. *(32:73)*

112. **(D)** The surgical scrub is the process of removing as many microorganisms from the hands and arms by mechanical washing and chemical antisepsis. *(2:124)*

113. **(D)** The arm is scrubbed, including the elbow and the antecubital space to 2 inches above the elbow. *(32:74)*

114. **(D)** A sterile person turns his back to a nonsterile person or area when passing. *(2:89)*

115. **(C)** Drapes should be carried to the OR table folded. To prevent them from coming in contact with unclean items in transport. *(2:231)*

116. **(B)** When draping a table, open the drape toward the front of the table first. *(23:133)*

117. **(C)** When handing the skin towels, go to the side of the table on which the surgeon is draping to avoid reaching over the nonsterile table. *(2:232)*

118. **(B)** If a drape is placed incorrectly it is discarded. The circulating nurse peels it from the table without contaminating other drapes or the operative site. *(2:231)*

119. **(D)** Draping is always done from a sterile area to an unsterile area, draping nearest first. *(33:103)*

120. **(B)** Skin over the site of a soft-tissue tumor should be handled gently because vigorous scrubbing could dislodge underlying tumor cells. *(2:474)*

121. **(B)** To minimize the risk of disseminating malignant tumor cells outside the operative area, some surgeons follow a special technique in which instruments in contact with tumor cells are discarded after use. *(2:474)*

122. **(A)** The cassette is enclosed with a sterile cover if it is to be used on the sterile field. One opens the cover by protecting the hands with a cuff as the circulator places the cassette into it. *(2:296)*

123. **(A)** The gown is removed first, then the gloves, in order to protect the forearm, hands, and clothing from contacting bacteria on the outer portion of the gown. Mask is removed after leaving the room and is handled only by the strings. *(32:82)*

124. **(D)** Renografin is a frequently used radiopaque contrast medium. *(2:293)*

125. **(A)** The postoperative complication of powder granulomata can result from powder that is not properly removed from gloves before surgery. This can be avoided by rinsing gloves before approaching the operative site. *(32:79)*

126. **(B)** Personnel should stand 6 feet or more from the patient and out of direct beam during exposure. *(2:296)*

127. **(D)** Vein ligation and stripping requires one setup whereas the others each require two. *(2:317–318, 329, 331, 339)*

128. **(A)** Separate setups are used in skin preparation of the recipient and donor sites. The donor site is scrubbed first. Items used in preparation of the recipient site must not be permitted to contaminate the donor site. The donor site should be scrubbed with a colorless antiseptic agent so the surgeon can evaluate the vascularity of the graft postoperatively.   *(2:225)*

129. **(C)** In drop technique, the contaminated instruments are discarded in a single basin. Gloves (and possibly gowns) are changed by the surgical team, and the incisional area is redraped with clean towels.
    (11:211)

130. **(B)** The drop technique utilizes fewer instruments and furniture than a clean-closure setup. However, the clean-closure setup provides a greater margin of safety.
    (11:210–211)

131. **(A)** The best method of floor care is to flood with detergent-disinfectant and then vacuum after each case. Machine cleaning is more effective than hand-mopping.   *(2:157)*

132. **(D)** Between surgical procedures, all linens from open packs, whether soiled or not, should be discarded in linen hamper bags. Wet linen should be placed in the center of the bundle to prevent soaking through to the outside of the bag.   *(32:88)*

133. **(B)** If disposable suction units are not used, decontaminate contents with disinfectant prior to hopper disposal. Wash the container and autoclave it before reuse.
    (2:155)

134. **(A)** If the washer-sterilizer and autoclave are not in an immediately adjacent room, the scrub nurse removes gown, covers tray with a clean towel, carries it to the utility room, and places it in the washer-sterilizer or autoclave there. The towel should be brought back to the room and discarded. OR attire should not be touched with either tray or towel.
    (2:155)

CHAPTER 4

Supplies and Equipment
Questions

Directions: Each of the questions or incomplete statements below is followed by four suggested answers or completions. Select the best answer in each case.

A. SUTURES AND NEEDLES—CLASSIFICATION

1. Which suture loses much of its tensile strength after about 1 year in the body and usually disappears after a period of time?

A. polypropylene
B. stainless steel
C. nylon
D. silk

2. Next to stainless steel, the strongest nonabsorbable suture material is

A. polyester
B. nylon
C. polyglycolic acid
D. polyethylene

3. Silk, polyester, and nylon are sometimes coated in order to

A. make them easier to handle
B. reduce tissue reaction
C. prevent slippage
D. increase capillarity

4. The suture that causes the least reaction is

A. stainless steel
B. silk
C. nylon
D. cotton

5. A nonabsorbable suture with excellent handling qualities is

A. cotton
B. stainless steel
C. nylon
D. silk

6. Which suture has inconsistent tensile strength and knot security?

A. silk
B. surgical gut
C. polyester
D. cotton

7. A suture used in heart surgery because it has a high flex life is

A. collagen suture
B. polyglycolic acid suture
C. dermal silk suture
D. polyester suture

8. Why is nonabsorbable suture contraindicated around the kidney or ureter?

A. infection
B. stone formation
C. allergic response
D. absorption time

9. A needle with three sharp cutting tips at the points is classified as a

A. trocar
B. side cutting
C. reverse cutting
D. conventional cutting

10. The needle point used primarily in ophthalmic surgery is

A. taper point
B. trocar point
C. reverse cutting point
D. side cutting point

11.   The type of needle point used on tissue such as peritoneum and intestines is

A. taper point
B. blunt point
C. cutting point
D. trocar point

12.   The type of needle point used to suture friable tissue, such as liver and kidney, is a

A. side cutting point
B. trocar point
C. blunt point
D. cutting point

13.   All of the following are needles with a slit from the inside of the eye to the end of the needle through which a suture strand is drawn *except* a

A. French eye needle
B. spring eye needle
C. split eye needle
D. Mayo needle

14.   Which anatomic tissue would contradict the use of a cutting needle?

A. fascia
B. nerve
C. tendon
D. cervix

15.   When placing a swaged needle on a needle holder, clamp the needle holder

A. on the swaged area
B. on the tightest ratchet
C. about one-third down from the swage
D. with the needle close to the ratchet

16.   Which suture is inert in tissue, has high tensile strength, and gives support to a wound indefinitely?

A. nylon
B. silk
C. stainless steel
D. cotton

17.   Surgical gut is made from

A. submucosa of cat intestines
B. peritoneum of calves
C. submucosa of sheep intestines
D. peritoneum of beef animal

18.   Which type of suture would be used to invert the stump of an appendix?

A. buried
B. purse-string
C. mattress
D. tension

19.   A suture used to hold a structure to the side of the operative field is called a

A. traction suture
B. retention suture
C. stay suture
D. tension suture

20.   Each of the following is a coating for polyester sutures *except*

A. polybutilate
B. silicone
C. Teflon
D. polyamide polymer

21.   An acrylic, cementlike substance commonly referred to as bone cement is

A. polytetrafluoroethylene
B. polybutilate
C. glycoside
D. methyl methacrylate

22.   An aneurysm needle is used to

A. ligate a deep, large vessel
B. suction out fluid from an aneurysm
C. suture an aneurysm closed
D. inject the vascular system for x-ray study

23.   A continuous suture placed beneath the epithelial layer of the skin in short lateral stitches is called a

A. mattress suture
B. buried suture
C. retention suture
D. subcuticular suture

24.   A drawback to the use of steel suture is that it

A. breaks easily
B. is irritating to tissue
C. is difficult to handle
D. may be used in the presence of infection

25.   Plain surgical gut

A. is digested relatively quickly in the body
B. is treated with a salt solution to resist absorption
C. is used when the wound will be subjected to tension during healing
D. is a true, nonabsorbable material

26.   Which statement regarding synthetic absorbable polymer sutures is *not* true?

A. sutures are packaged dry
B. sutures are dipped in water before being handed to the surgeon
C. sutures produce only a mild tissue reaction during absorption
D. sutures are multifilamented

27. All of the following have a weakening effect on gut suture *except*

A. handling gut in a dry condition
B. straightening gut after it has dried
C. storing gut in a dry towel before handing it to the surgeon
D. running gloved fingers down the strand while straightening it

28. Why is silk not recommended for use in urinary or biliary surgery?

A. it may become the nucleus for stone formation
B. it lacks elasticity
C. it is decomposed by urine and bile
D. it is not strong enough

29. Tissue trauma is best minimized by using a

A. threaded suture on a taper needle
B. threaded suture on a cutting needle
C. suture swaged on a needle
D. suture threaded on a spring-eye needle

30. Why are bumpers or bolsters used on retention sutures?

A. to prevent the suture from cutting into the skin surface
B. to facilitate easy removal
C. to identify the order of suture removal
D. to prevent unequal tension on the wound edges

31. The man who advocated the principles of meticulous hemostasis, the use of silk sutures, and the elimination of dead spaces was

A. William Halsted
B. Ambroise Paré
C. Philip Physick
D. Johns Hopkins

32. A tissue repair material that increases the amount of tissue already present and becomes a living part of the tissue it supports is

A. polyester fiber mesh
B. cargile membrane
C. polypropylene mesh
D. fascia lata

33. Ligatures are used to

A. prevent evisceration
B. occlude the lumen of a blood vessel
C. bring tissue together
D. hold tissues together until healing takes place

34. The measure of how much pull a suture can withstand before it will break is called

A. yield power

B. tensile strength
C. capillarity
D. gauge

35. If infection is present, surgical gut is

A. absorbed more rapidly
B. absorbed less rapidly
C. absorbed at the same rate
D. not absorbed

36. A nonabsorbable synthetic suture that is strong, least reactive in tissue, and used widely in cardiovascular procedures is

A. nylon suture
B. polypropylene suture
C. polyglycolic acid suture
D. dermal silk

37. Which suture would be used on an aortic valve replacement?

A. polypropolene
B. vicryl
C. dermalon
D. dexon

38. Which statement concerning silk suture is false?

A. silk is an animal product
B. silk causes less tissue reaction than surgical gut
C. silk stays in the body permanently
D. silk loses its tensile strength when moistened

39. Suture that must be moistened before it is handed to the surgeon in order to increase its tensile strength is

A. silk
B. polyester
C. plain surgical gut
D. cotton

40. A suture widely used in tendon repair is

A. nylon
B. polyglycolic acid
C. stainless steel
D. collagen

B. INSTRUMENTS—CLASSIFICATION

41. Spinal fusion setups require

A. Cottle elevators
B. Doyen elevators
C. Cobb elevators
D. Lempert elevators

42. Which instrument is necessary in effecting a cholecystostomy?

A. Lahey gall duct forceps
B. Mayo cystic duct scoop
C. Ochsner gallbladder trocar
D. Randall stone forceps

43. Which blade is indicated for use on a #4 knife handle?

A. 10
B. 11
C. 15
D. 20

44. The suction appropriate for use in deep abdominal irrigation is

A. Yankauer
B. Poole
C. Adson
D. Frazier

45. A solid knife used to cut the sternum during chest surgery is

A. Langenbeck
B. Lebsche
C. Hurd
D. Lambert-Berry

46. A small, spring-type peripheral vascular clamp is a

A. DeBakey
B. Potts bulldog
C. Satinsky
D. Jackson

47. Which of the following instruments is *not* an example of a rongeur?

A. Kerrison
B. Hudson
C. Leksell
D. Lempert

48. An adapter to the Hall air driver necessary for screw insertion is the

A. Jacobs' chuck
B. Trinkle chuck
C. reciprocating head
D. 500 rpm Hall head

49. Kerrison refers to a/an

A. elevator
B. retractor
C. rongeur
D. rasp

50. Weitlaner refers to a

A. retractor
B. forceps
C. bone holder
D. bone cutter

51. Which item is a bone holder?

A. Stille-Leur
B. Lane
C. Cobb
D. Ruchin

52. What surgical specialty utilizes Hibbs retractors?

A. vascular
B. ophthalmology
C. orthopedics
D. rectal

53. Which needle holder would be used in open-heart surgery?

A. Castroviejo
B. Heaney
C. Webster
D. Ayer

54. Which of the following instruments would *not* be found on a resection and recession?

A. Jameson muscle hook
B. Castroviejo caliper
C. Castroviejo trephine
D. Stevens scissor

55. A self-retaining neurosurgical retractor that is used in maintaining traction on brain tissue is the

A. Beckman-Adson
B. Cloward
C. Leyla-Yasargil
D. Jansen

56. A Freer is a/an

A. scissor
B. retractor
C. forceps
D. elevator

57. Which of the following instruments is *not* a nasal septum forceps?

A. McCoy
B. Ballinger
C. Asch
D. Bruening

58. Ferguson-Frazier refers to a

A. retractor
B. suction
C. scissor
D. grasper

59. What instrument would be used to enlarge the burr hole made during a craniotomy?

A. rongeur
B. periosteal elevator
C. Gigli saw
D. Cloward punch

60. In what type of surgery is a Lowman used?

A. orthopedic
B. plastic
C. ophthalmic
D. thoracic

61. Which instrument has no teeth?

A. Allis
B. Kelly
C. Kocher
D. Jacobs

62. Wescott scissors are used in

A. plastic surgery
B. ophthalmic surgery
C. vascular surgery
D. orthopedic surgery

63. In which procedure would a Murphy-Lane bone skid be used?

A. laminectomy
B. meniscectomy
C. hip prosthesis
D. Bankart procedure

64. Biting of small pieces of soft tissue during neurosurgical procedures requires the use of a

A. Kerrison rongeur
B. Leksell rongeur
C. Cushing rongeur
D. Stille-Luer rongeur

65. Which instrument is not always required in the insertion of compression screws?

A. power drill
B. depth gauge
C. chuck key
D. metal ruler

66. Which of the following is *not* a bowel resection clamp?

A. Dennis
B. Allen
C. Duval
D. DeMartel

67. Which instrument would be used in a splenectomy?

A. Doyen
B. Allen
C. Jacobs
D. pedicle clamp

68. A Sheeley ossicle forceps is used in

A. ophthalmic surgery
B. ear surgery
C. vascular surgery
D. orthopedic surgery

69. Lacrimal probes are

A. Bakes
B. Bowman
C. Van Buren
D. Hegar

70. Hegenbarth clip-applying forceps aid in the application of

A. Heifitz clips
B. Raney clips
C. Scoville clips
D. Michel clips

71. Which scissor is used for heavy dissection?

A. Wescott
B. Potts-Smith
C. curved Mayo
D. Metzenbaum

72. A Hurd pillar retractor is used for

A. appendectomy
B. plastic surgery
C. nasal surgery
D. tonsillectomy

73. An adenotome is a

A. retractor
B. curette
C. dissector
D. grasper

74. An elevator used in ear surgery is a

A. McKentry
B. Love-Adson
C. Lempert
D. Hibbs

75. A Taylor retractor is used in a

A. total hip replacement
B. meniscectomy
C. laminectomy
D. hip nailing

76. A Bailey is a

A. retractor
B. rongeur
C. dissecting forceps
D. rib approximator

77. A Bethune is a/an

A. elevator
B. raspatory
C. rib shear
D. rongeur

78. Which speculum is used in nasal surgery?

A. Lancaster
B. Maumeneek-Park
C. Pratt
D. Killian

79. An Auvard is a

A. forceps
B. dissector
C. speculum
D. sound

80. A Parker is a

A. grasper
B. dissector
C. retractor
D. hemostat

81. A Freer is a/an

A. elevator
B. nerve hook
C. forceps
D. speculum

82. What coating substance is used in the surgical instrument manufacturing process to make instruments more corrosion resistant?

A. nucleic acid
B. nitric acid
C. Rustoleum
D. instrument milk

83. A curved forceps with fenestrated blades and no teeth, which grips or encloses delicate structures such as a ureter or a fallopian tube is a

A. Hibbs
B. Babcock
C. Lahey
D. Crile

C. DRESSINGS AND PACKINGS

84. A sponge used in brain surgery is a/an

A. cottonoid patty
B. Kitner
C. impregnated gauze
D. porcine

85. Once the peritoneum is entered, which of the following procedures is *not* acceptable?

A. remove all free sponges from the field
B. use 4-by-4 sponges on sponge forceps only
C. give free sponges to the surgeon only on an exchange basis
D. keep a mental count of free sponges on the field

86. Seamless tubular cotton that stretches to fit a contour and is used for padding is called

A. Ace bandage
B. Webril
C. sheet wadding
D. stockingette

87. What is the proper wrapping procedure utilizing an Esmarch bandage?

A. start at the distal end of the extremity
B. start at the proximal end of the extremity
C. start after the cuff is inflated
D. A or B

88. What is the purpose of using warm laparotomy pads?

A. to control capillary bleeding
B. to hasten clotting
C. to decrease the need for oxygen to the tissues
D. A or B

89. An item used for padding that has smooth and clingy layers is called

A. Webril
B. stockingette
C. Telfa
D. gypsum

90. Rectal packing is made of petroleum-treated gauze in order to

A. aid in packing removal
B. facilitate easier bowel movement
C. effect rectal hemostasis
D. prevent postoperative infection

91. An elastic adhesive bandage is

A. flexible collodian
B. Ace bandage
C. elastoplast
D. scultetus binder

92. Montgomery straps are used to

A. secure head dressings
B. hold a thyroid dressing in place
C. conform a dressing to body structures
D. hold in place bulky dressings that require frequent changing

93. A dissecting sponge that is a small roll of heavy cotton tape is a

A. Kitner
B. peanut
C. tonsil
D. tape

94. A dissecting sponge made of gauze that is used to dissect or absorb fluid is called a

A. patty
B. tonsil
C. cottonoid
D. peanut

95. A temporary biologic dressing is

A. porcine
B. Telfa
C. collagen
D. mesh

96. Which procedure would *not* require a pressure dressing?

A. plastic surgery
B. knee surgery
C. radical mastectomy
D. hysterectomy

97. A sponge that is cotton-filled gauze with a cotton thread attached is a

A. patty
B. tonsil
C. Kitner
D. peanut

98. Patties are

A. used dry
B. moistened with saline
C. moistened with water
D. moistened with silver nitrate solution

99. Lap pads or tapes are used

A. dry
B. moistened with saline
C. moistened with water
D. B or C

100. Which is *not* a reason for a pressure dressing?

A. prevents edema

B. conforms to body contour
C. absorbs extensive drainage
D. distributes pressure evenly

101. Which of the following can be a supplement to a subcuticular closure?

A. skin staples
B. swaged sutures
C. stent fixation
D. skin closure tapes

102. A protective skin coating is accomplished with

A. tincture of benzoin
B. merthiolate
C. iodoform
D. Lugol's solution

103. Which of the following is a nonadhesive dressing?

A. collodian
B. elastoplast
C. kling
D. adaptic

D. CATHETERS, DRAINS, TUBES, AND COLLECTING MECHANISMS

104. The smallest diameter on a French scale is a

A. 3
B. 5
C. 7
D. 9

105. How much sterile water is needed to properly inflate a 5-cc balloon of a Foley catheter?

A. 3 ml
B. 5 ml
C. 6 ml
D. 10 ml

106. A double-lumen gastrointestinal tube is called a

A. Harris
B. Cantor
C. Miller-Abbott
D. Levin

107. A single-lumen mercury-weighted gastrointestinal tube with a lumen of 14 French is a

A. Miller-Abbott
B. Harris
C. Levin
D. Cantor

108. A 10-foot, No. 18 French gastrointestinal tube with a mercury-filled bag at its extreme end is called a

A. Levin
B. Miller-Abbott
C. Harris
D. Cantor

109. What type of catheter would facilitate the removal of small gallstones?

A. T tube
B. Robinson
C. Fogarty
D. Rehfus

110. In which procedure could a Fogarty catheter be utilized?

A. embolectomy
B. gastrectomy
C. craniotomy
D. thorocotomy

111. A tube used in the emergency control of hemorrhage from bleeding esophageal varices is called a

A. Rehfus
B. Cantor
C. Miller-Abbott
D. Sengstaken-Blakemore

112. A catheter commonly used in a gastrostomy is a

A. mushroom
B. Rehfus
C. Cantor
D. Sengstaken-Blakemore

113. What drain would commonly be used in a radical neck dissection?

A. Penrose
B. rubber tissue
C. water-seal
D. Hemovac

114. A drain that is widely used to facilitate the escape of fluid from a wound is the

A. sump
B. Penrose
C. water-seal
D. Foley

115. Which of the following is *not* a type of ureteral catheter tip?

A. whistle
B. olive
C. Braasch bulb
D. Pezzar

116. Which is *not* a basket-type stone dislodger?

A. Dormia
B. Gibbons
C. Johnson
D. Levant

117. Which ureteral catheter is used to dilate the ureter?

A. Garceau tapered tip
B. basket catheter
C. flexible filiform tip
D. stent

118. All of the following statements are true of ureteral catheters *except* that they

A. are made of flexible woven nylon or plastic
B. range in caliber from size 3 to 14 French
C. have graduated markings
D. provide direct visualization of the bladder

119. Before handing a Penrose drain to the surgeon,

A. place it on an Allis clamp
B. attach a safety pin to it
C. cut it to the desired length
D. moisten it in saline

120. A drain with a strip of gauze on its inside is called a

A. sump drain
B. vessel-loop
C. cigarette drain
D. rubber dam

121. Tubular structures are commonly drained with a

A. Cantor
B. T tube
C. Hemovac
D. Penrose

122. A stone basket is used to remove ureteral calculi in

A. the upper third of the ureter
B. any portion of the ureter
C. the lower third of the ureter
D. the ureteral orifice only

123. A central venous pressure catheter is usually inserted into the

A. brachial vein
B. cephalic vein
C. femoral vein
D. subclavian vein

124. When drawing a blood sample, what is considered a safe time lapse between blood drawing and analysis?

A. 10 minutes
B. 20 minutes
C. 30 minutes
D. 1 hour

125. What is a potential hazard to the patient when using a cardiac catheter?

A. electrocution
B. burns
C. incompatibility
D. allergic response

126. Which of the following is *not* used for urethral dilation?

A. bougie
B. metal sound
C. Hegar dilator
D. filliform and follower

127. A closed-wound suction system works by

A. positive pressure
B. negative-pressure vacuum
C. air displacement
D. constant gravity drainage

128. Why is a 30-cc bag Foley used after a TUR of the prostate?

A. hemostasis
B. decompression
C. creation of negative pressure
D. aspiration

129. The tube that collects bronchial washings is

A. Broyles
B. Luki
C. Ellik
D. Toomey

130. To which mechanical vacuum suction pump is a Levin tube often attached?

A. Sachs suction
B. Adson suction
C. Gomco suction
D. Stern-McCarthy

131. A Pezzar is a/an

A. Foley catheter
B. bat-wing catheter
C. ureteral catheter
D. mushroom catheter

132. A type of nasogastric tube is a

A. Wangansteen
B. Miller-Abbott
C. Yankauer
D. Ferguson-Frazier

133. The three lumens of a Foley are used for inflation, drainage, and

A. prevention of urine reflux
B. access for sterile urine specimens
C. continuous irrigation
D. additional hemostasis

E. EQUIPMENT

134. An image intensifier

A. is an x-ray machine
B. is a microscope
C. converts the x-ray beam into a fluoroscopic optical image
D. converts an x-ray image into film

135. Extracorporeal circulation refers to circulation

A. of blood outside of the body
B. through the muscular tissue of the heart
C. established through an anastomosis between two vessels
D. of blood through the whole body except the lungs

136. The scoring system that assesses an infant's condition after birth is called a/an

A. Roentgen
B. Romberg
C. Apgar
D. colostrum

137. Which procedure records the electrical activity of the brain?

A. electrocardiogram
B. brain scan
C. electromyogram
D. electroencephalogram

138. Which of the following can assist in locating a metallic foreign body?

A. Berman
B. Smith
C. Ferguson
D. Jones

139. A unit for describing an exposure dose of radiation is a/an

A. Romberg's sign
B. ROP
C. roentgen
D. rostrum

140. A grounding pad is *not* required for the electrocautery in

A. a cutting current setting
B. a coagulation current setting
C. a monopolar unit
D. a bipolar unit

141. Which dermatome limits the length of the graft obtained?

A. Brown
B. Hall
C. skin-graft knife
D. Reese

142. Which graft must be obtained with a dermatome?

A. split-thickness meshgraft
B. full-thickness Wolfe graft
C. free myocutaneous graft
D. full-thickness pinch graft

143. Use of the microscope during surgery magnifies the surgical field by

A. 2x–2.8x
B. 6x–40x
C. 20x–100x
D. 50x–100x

144. The proper setting for a tourniquet applied to an arm is

A. 100–200 mm Hg
B. 250–300 mm Hg
C. 350–450 mm Hg
D. 400–500 mm Hg

145. All of the following are attachments to the 3M mini-driver *except* the

A. Swanson reamer chuck
B. Jacobs drill chuck
C. oscillating saw chuck
D. sagittal saw chuck

146. Adapting a Hall air-driver for drill bit insertion requires the addition of a

A. Trinkle chuck
B. Jacobs chuck
C. Swanson chuck
D. K-wire driver

147. Ernst appliances are used to

A. provide birth control
B. prevent postoperative hemorrhage
C. effect uterine evacuation
D. insert radium

148. A Cavitron unit is used for

A. cyclodialysis
B. photocoagulation
C. phacoemulsification
D. cryotherapy

149. The power source for Hall power equipment is

A. carbon dioxide
B. nitrous oxide
C. nitrogen
D. electricity

150. The Waters' perfusion machine is used for

A. open-heart surgery
B. kidney transplants
C. hemodialysis
D. peritoneal dialysis

151. An air-powered instrument useful in spinal procedures is the

A. Ronjair
B. Neurairtome
C. Surgairtome
D. Light-Veley

152. In cardiopulmonary bypass surgery, a pump oxygenator is used. The oxygenator

A. simulates the pumping action of the right ventricle
B. measures venous pressure
C. adds additional oxygen to the heart
D. simulates the function of the lungs

153. In the pump oxygenator used in cardiopulmonary bypass, the pump portion simulates the pumping action of the

A. left ventricle
B. right ventricle
C. left atrium
D. right atrium

154. Air is introduced into the subarachnoid space via a lumbar puncture in order to visualize the ventricular and intercranial space of the brain in a/an

A. angiogram
B. myelogram
C. ventriculogram
D. pneumoencephalogram

155. Loupes are used for

A. tissue retraction
B. magnification
C. hemostasis
D. patient transfer

156. In electrocautery use, the inactive electrode

A. dispenses the current back to the unit
B. is an oscillating, low frequency electric current
C. freezes diseased tissue
D. is placed on the tissue by the surgeon

157. What radiographic procedure is used to insert endocardial electrodes?

A. ultrasound
B. image intensifier
C. angiography
D. arteriography

158. The fixed rate of pacing on an asynchronous model pacemaker is

A. 60 bpm
B. 72 bpm
C. 80 bpm
D. 84 bpm

159. What attachment to the craniotome is required to effect a bone flap after trephination?

A. 7 mm shell
B. neuroblade with dura guard
C. 12 mm shell perforator
D. wire-pass attachment

160. Which laser emission is primarily absorbed in tissue by hemoglobin or melanin?

A. CO_2
B. argon
C. Nd-YAG
D. helium-neon

Answers and Explanations

A. SUTURES AND NEEDLES—CLASSIFICATION

1. **(D)** Silk loses much of its tensile strength after 1 year and usually disappears after 2 or more years. Thus it is not a true nonabsorbable suture. *(2:257)*

2. **(A)** Polyester sutures are nonabsorbable synthetic sutures which are processed as multifilament braids. They are the strongest suture material except for stainless steel and they resist fraying and fragmentation. They are widely used in prosthetic devices because of their extended flex life. *(35:34)*

3. **(A)** Silk is treated with silicone or wax to make it easier for the suture to pass through tissue and facilitate knot tying. Polyester and braided nylon can be coated to increase the ease of handling for the surgeon. *(35:19)*

4. **(A)** Sutures that are inert do not readily interact chemically with tissues; thus they have low tissue reactivity. Stainless steel is the most inert suture material. *(35:23)*

5. **(D)** Silk is nonabsorbable. It is excellent for its handling qualities because it is flexible, smooth, and easy to tie. *(35:30)*

6. **(B)** Surgical gut is a strong suture material but its tensile strength is inconsistent. It also has inconsistent knot security. Gut is not as dependable as synthetic absorbables, which have predictable rates of absorption and tensile strength. *(35:28)*

7. **(D)** Flex life of a suture refers to its ability to bend without breaking. In heart surgery polyester suture can be used because of its high flex life. It is able to withstand the pumping action of the heart, which makes the suture bend continuously. *(35:21)*

8. **(B)** Surgical catgut is the suture of choice around the kidney and ureter because nonabsorbable suture can precipitate stone formation. *(17:118)*

9. **(A)** A trocar has sharp cutting tips at the points of a tapered needle. All three edges of the tip are sharpened to provide cutting action with the smallest possible hole in tissue as it penetrates. *(2:260)*

10. **(D)** A side cutting needle is relatively flat on top and bottom with angulated cutting edges on the sides. It is used primarily in ophthalmic surgery because it will not penetrate underlying tissue. It splits through the layer of tissue. *(2:260)*

11. **(A)** A taper point needle is used, on soft tissue, such as intestines and peritoneum, which offer a small amount of resistance to the needle as it passes through. *(2:260)*

12. **(C)** A rounded blunt point at the tip of a tapered needle is called a blunt point. It is used for suturing friable tissue, such as liver and kidney, because the blunt point will not cut through tissue. In this way the needle is less likely than a sharp-pointed needle to puncture a vessel in these organs. *(2:260)*

13. **(D)** A French eye needle, also referred to as a spring eye or split eye, has a slit from the inside of the eye to the end of the needle through which the suture strand is drawn. *(2:261)*

14. **(B)** Cutting edge needles are used on tough tissue, i.e., skin, fascia, tendon, cervix. Round tapered needles are used on nerve, peritoneum, muscle, lung, intestine, and dura mater. *(2:263)*

15. **(C)** The correct position of a curved needle in a needle holder is about one-third down from the swage. The needle is placed securely in the tip of the needle holder jaws and closed on the first or second ratchet.   *(2:262)*

16. **(C)** Surgical steel is inert in tissue, has high tensile strength, and gives the greatest strength of any suture material to a wound before healing begins. It supports a wound indefinitely.   *(2:258)*

17. **(C)** Surgical gut is collagen derived from the submucosa of sheep intestine and of the serosa of beef intestine.   *(2:256)*

18. **(B)** A purse-string suture is a continuous suture placed around a lumen and tightened, drawstring fashion, to close the lumen. This is used, for example, when inverting the stump of an appendix or when closing the anus in the perineal stage of an abdominoperineal resection.   *(2:262, 329)*

19. **(A)** A traction suture holds a structure out of the way by retracting it to the side of the operative field, such as the tongue in a mouth operation. Usually a nonabsorbable suture is used.   *(2:263)*

20. **(D)** Polybutilate, silicone, and polytetrafluoroethylene, known by the DuPont trade name of Teflon, are used to coat polyester fiber suture to lubricate the surfaces for a smooth passage through tissue.   *(2:259)*

21. **(D)** Bone cement is methyl methacrylate. It is recommended that ORs provide a suitable exhaust system to collect the vapors as it is mixed in order to reduce inhalation of the potentially hazardous fumes.   *(2:267)*

22. **(A)** An aneurysm needle is an instrument with a blunt needle on the end. The eye is on the distal end of the needle. The needles are made symmetrically right and left. The surgeon uses them to take a ligature around a deep, large vessel, as in a thyroidectomy or in thoracic surgery.   *(2:263)*

23. **(D)** A subcuticular suture is a continuous suture placed beneath the epithelial layer of the skin in short lateral stitches. It leaves a minimal scar.   *(2:262–263)*

24. **(C)** Stainless steel is inert in tissue, very strong, and can be used in the presence of infection, however it lacks elasticity and is hard to handle and knot.   *(2:258)*

25. **(A)** Plain surgical gut is digested relatively quickly, usually in 5 to 10 days. It is used to ligate small vessels and to suture subcutaneous fat. However, it is not used to suture layers likely to be subjected to tension during healing.   *(2:256)*

26. **(B)** Sutures are packaged and used dry. They should not be soaked or dipped in water or saline as this may reduce the tensile strength of the suture.   *(2:257)*

27. **(C)** Straightened gut may be stored between the folds of a dry sterile towel if it must be prepared in advance. The dry gut may be moistened in cool sterile water or saline for no more than 4 to 6 seconds just before handing to the surgeon. Ideally, the suture should remain in its original packet as long as possible in order to best preserve its good handling properties.   *(35:48, 49)*

28. **(A)** Foreign bodies in the presence of fluids containing high concentrations of crystalloids may act as a nucleus for precipitation and stone formation. This is why, in the urinary and biliary tract, rapidly absorbed sutures are used.   *(15:28)*

29. **(C)** A swaged-on needle provides a smooth juncture between material and needle, thus creating a smaller hole than threaded eyed needles make. Tissue trauma and oozing are minimized.   *(35:52–53)*

30. **(A)** A bumper is passed over or through the exposed portion of suture in a retention suture in order to prevent the suture from cutting into the skin surface.   *(32:110)*

31. **(A)** Dr. William Halsted advocated the principles of meticulous hemostasis, the use of fine interrupted silk sutures consistent with the strength of the tissues to be sutured, cutting knot ends close to the knot, and the elimination of dead spaces by proper tissue approximation.   *(35:81)*

32. **(D)** Fascia lata contains collagen and becomes a living part of the tissue it supports.   *(2:267)*

33. **(B)** A ligature or tie is a suture material tied around a blood vessel to occlude the lumen.   *(2:254)*

34. **(B)** Tensile strength is the measured pounds of tension or pull that a strand will withstand before it breaks.   *(2:254)*

35. **(A)** Surgical gut can be used in the presence of infection; however, absorption takes place much more rapidly if infection is present.   *(2:256)*

36. **(B)** Polypropylene is strong, essentially nonreactive, and is used in the instances where suture must be left in place for a long time. It can be used in the presence of infection. It has become a choice material for cardiovascular procedures because of its smooth passage through tissue as well as its strength and inertness.   *(2:259)*

37. **(A)** In aortic valve replacement, the aortotomy is closed with continuous prolene (polypropolene) which is a nonabsorbable suture.   *(17:382, 118)*

38. **(C)** Silk is not a true nonabsorbable suture. It loses much of its tensile strength after about 1 year and usually disappears after 2 or more years.   *(2:257)*

39. **(D)** Cotton is one of the weakest of the nonabsorbable materials. However, it gains tensile strength when wet; for this reason it is moistened before being handed to the surgeon.   *(2:257)*

40. **(C)** Stainless steel has high tensile strength, gives great strength to a wound, and supports a wound indefinitely. It is widely used in the respiratory tract, in tendon repair, and for general wound closure.   *(2:258)*

B. INSTRUMENTS—CLASSIFICATION

41. **(C)** A set of Cobb elevators is required on all spinal fusions.   *(6:192)*

42. **(C)** An Ochsner gallbladder trocar is necessary for the drainage of an inflamed gallbladder.   *(32:187)*

43. **(D)** A #4 knife handle holds both a #20 and #22 blade. A #3 knife handle and a #7 knife handle hold a #10, #15, #11, and #12 blade.   *(32:143)*

44. **(B)** Poole suction is used effectively when attempting to suction gross amounts of fluids.   *(32:147)*

45. **(B)** A Lebsche sternum knife is used in chest surgery to open the sternum in an anterior procedure.   *(32:361)*

46. **(B)** The Potts bulldog clamp is a small, peripheral vascular spring-operated clamp. They are angled, straight, or curved.   *(6:247)*

47. **(B)** The Hudson is a hand drill used to create burr holes.   *(32:726)*

48. **(B)** The Trinkle chuck for automatic screwdriver attachment is a valuable attachment to the Hall air driver and is necessary for screw insertion.   *(6:176)*

49. **(C)** Kerrison refers to a rongeur. It is available in many angles and is used extensively in surgery of the spine and neurosurgery.   *(6:188)*

50. **(A)** Weitlaner is a self-retaining rake retractor.   *(6:28)*

51. **(B)** Lane is a bone holder used for holding bone shafts.   *(6:116)*

52. **(C)** Hibbs are double-ended retractors used in orthopedic surgery. They are available in graduated sizes.   *(6:115)*

53. **(A)** A Castroviejo needle holder is indicated in open-heart surgery.   *(6:275)*

54. **(C)** A Castroviejo trephine would be used to remove a cornea in a keratoplasty. The other instruments are used to perform a resection and recession.   *(32:677)*

55. **(C)** When used in combination with delicate malleable brain spatulas, the Leyla-Yasargil provides ease in retraction of brain tissue.   *(32:743)*

56. **(D)** A Freer is a fine, double-ended elevator. It may be curved or straight and is used extensively in all delicate surgery.   *(6:255, 396)*

57. **(B)** Ballinger refers to a swivel knife or a nasal gouge. McCoy, Asch, and Bruening are all septum cutting forceps.   *(32:617, 618)*

58. **(B)** Ferguson-Frazier suction is available in several sizes. It is used in ENT, vascular, plastic, and neurosurgery.   *(32:541, 727)*

59. **(A)** Additional bone may be removed with a rongeur to increase exposure of the brain.   *(2:434)*

60. **(A)** A Lowman is a bone-holding forceps used in orthopedics. It is a self-retaining bone clamp.   *(32:491)*

61. **(B)** A Kelly clamp is serrated for adequate hemostasis without tissue trauma. It is used to secure larger areas than those served by the Halstead or Crile clamp.   *(6:15)*

62. **(B)** Wescott scissors are fine, blunt scissors with a spring action. They are used in ophthalmic surgery.   *(6:375)*

63. **(C)** The Murphy-Lane bone skid is used extensively in hip prosthesis, including total hip replacement.   *(6:149)*

64. **(C)** The Cushing rongeur is an angled scissor-type rongeur useful in biting small bits of soft tissue during neurosurgery.   *(6:441)*

65. **(A)** Power is not necessary for insertion of compression screws. A hand drill may be used along with a metal ruler, a depth gauge, and chuck key for removal of drill bits.   *(6:167)*

66. **(C)** The Duval is a lung-grasping forceps used only in thoracic procedures. The Allen and DeMartel are anastomosis clamps and the Dennis is an intestinal forceps.   *(32:211)*

67. **(D)** For splenectomy, prepare a basic laparotomy set plus two large right-angled pedicle clamps and long instruments. *(32:304)*

68. **(B)** The malleus, incus, and stapes are the ossicles of the middle ear. The Sheehey ossicle forceps is used in delicate ear surgery. *(6:349)*

69. **(D)** Bowman probes are used to probe the lacrimal duct in a dacryocystorhinostomy. *(6:411)*

70. **(D)** Michel clips are available on a wire rack and are loaded into Hengenbarth appliers for use by the scrub person. *(6:432)*

71. **(C)** The Mayo scissor, both curved and straight, may be used for heavy tissue dissection. All of the others are fine tissue dissectors. *(32:116)*

72. **(D)** A pillar retractor is used during a tonsillectomy to stabilize the tonsil at its pillar attachment for final dissection of the tonsil. The opposite end of the retractor is a dissector which is used to free the tonsil. *(32:637)*

73. **(C)** An adenotome is a short, guillotine blade-like dissector used to remove adenoids. *(6:320)*

74. **(C)** The Lempert elevator is used in delicate ear surgery. The Hibbs and Love-Adson are heavy orthopedic periosteal elevators. The McKentry is used in nasal surgery. *(6:347)*

75. **(C)** The Taylor retractor is a spinal retractor used in a laminectomy. *(6:184)*

76. **(D)** The Bailey rib approximator is used to approximate the ribs for closure of a thoracic incision prior to closure of the chest with heavy chromic suture. *(6:236)*

77. **(C)** The Bethune rib shear is used in thoracic surgery to sever the rib from its anterior and posterior attachments before placement of the Finoshietto retractor. *(6:238)*

78. **(D)** The Killian septum speculum is used in nasal surgery. *(6:290)*

79. **(C)** An Auvard is a speculum that is weighted for use in the vaginal tract. *(32:326)*

80. **(C)** The Parker retractor is a small double-ended retractor for superficial tissue retraction. *(6:36)*

81. **(A)** A Freer elevator is used extensively in ENT, neurosurgery, and fine orthopedic procedures. *(32:626)*

82. **(B)** Instruments go through a passivation process by being placed in nitric acid to remove any residue of carbon steel. The nitric acid also produces a surface coating of chromium oxide. Chromium oxide provides a resistance to corrosion. *(32:115)*

83. **(B)** A Babcock forceps is a curved fenestrated blade clamp with no teeth that grasps or encloses delicate structures such as ureter, appendix, or fallopian tube. *(32:117)*

C. DRESSING AND PACKINGS

84. **(A)** Cottonoid patties are compressed rayon or cotton sponges that are used moist on delicate structures such as nerves, brain, and spinal cord. *(2:138)*

85. **(D)** Once the peritoneum is opened or the incision extends deep into a body cavity, the following precautions must be taken: Remove all small sponges from the field and use only tapes, use 4-by-4 sponges on sponge forceps only, and give sponges to the surgeon one at a time on an exchange basis. *(2:152)*

86. **(D)** Stockingette is a knitted, seamless tubing of cotton 1 to 12 inches wide. It stretches to fit any contour snugly. *(2:377)*

87. **(A)** Wrapping of an extremity begins at the distal end. *(2:250)*

88. **(D)** Hot packs are frequently impacted into extensive wounds to control capillary bleeding. The addition of heat accelerates the natural chemical reaction of the blood to hasten clotting. *(2:253)*

89. **(A)** Webril is a soft, lint-free cotton bandage. The surface is smooth but not glazed, so that each layer clings to the preceding one and the padding lies smoothly in place. *(2:377)*

90. **(A)** The first dressing change following anal surgery may be very painful; therefore, it is well to protect the edges of wounds with petroleum gauze. *(2:584–585)*

91. **(C)** This bandage is preferable for holding dressings in place over mobile areas such as the neck or extremities, or where pressure is required. *(7:364)*

92. **(D)** Montgomery straps are used to hold in place bulky dressings that require frequent changes or wound inspections. They are made in pairs, in assorted widths, with strings. One strap is put on each side of the dressing and the strings are tied across the dressing. *(2:149)*

93. **(A)** Kitner dissecting sponges are small rolls of heavy cotton tape which are held in forceps. *(2:138)*

94. **(D)** Peanut sponges are very small gauze sponges used to dissect or absorb fluid in delicate procedures.
(2:138)

95. **(A)** Pig skin (porcine) is used as a temporary biologic dressing to cover large body surfaces denuded of skin.
(2:269)

96. **(D)** Pressure dressings are used frequently following extensive operations, especially in plastic surgery, knee operations, and radical mastectomies.   *(2:142)*

97. **(B)** Tonsil sponges are cotton-filled gauze with a cotton thread attached.   *(2:138)*

98. **(B)** Patties are moistened with saline and pressed out flat on a metal surface. They could pick up lint if placed on a towel.   *(2:431)*

99. **(B)** Normal saline is usually used to moisten sponges and tapes because it is an isotonic solution.   *(2:141)*

100. **(B)** A pressure dressing prevents edema, distributes pressure evenly, absorbs excessive drainage, gives extra wound support, and provides comfort to the patient post-op.   *(2:142)*

101. **(D)** Skin closure tapes may be used instead of or supplementary to closure if very close approximation of skin is required for good cosmetic results.   *(2:445)*

102. **(A)** Tincture of benzoin is a protective coating substance which is frequently applied to the skin before adhesive dressings are used.   *(35:192)*

103. **(D)** Adaptic is a nonadherent surgical dressing placed over the suture line. The other materials that make up the dressing are prevented from adhering to the incision.   *(17:112)*

D. CATHETERS, DRAINS, TUBES, AND COLLECTING MECHANISMS

104. **(A)** Instruments and catheters are measured on a French scale; the diameter (in millimeters) is multiplied by 3. The smallest is 1 mm in diameter times 3, or 3 French.   *(2:262)*

105. **(D)** Ten ml of sterile water are needed to properly inflate a 5-cc balloon to compensate for the volume required by the inflation channel.   *(2:221)*

106. **(C)** The Miller-Abbott is a double-lumen, No. 16 French tube, one lumen of which is used to introduce mercury or inflate the balloon at the end of the tube; the other, entirely independent, is used for aspiration. Markings on the tube indicate the distance it has been passed.
(7:725)

107. **(B)** A Harris tube is a single-lumen mercury-weighted tube about 6 feet long with a lumen of 14 on the French scale. It has a metal tip and is used for suction and irrigation. The weight of the mercury carries the bag by gravity.   *(7:725)*

108. **(D)** The Cantor tube is 10 feet long and No. 18 French. Its distinguishing features are that it is larger and has a mercury-filled bag at the extreme end of the rubber tubing.   *(7:725)*

109. **(C)** A Fogarty-type biliary catheter is a balloon-tipped catheter used to facilitate the removal of small stones and debris in the duct of the gallbladder.   *(32:188)*

110. **(A)** In an embolectomy, a Fogarty catheter is inserted beyond the point of clot attachment. The balloon is inflated and the catheter is withdrawn along with the detached clot.   *(32:434)*

111. **(D)** Esophageal varices are treated with a compressing double-balloon tube which acts as a tamponade. It should be chilled and lubricated before passing. One balloon is inflated in the stomach and one in the esophagus.   *(7:822)*

112. **(A)** Mushroom catheters and Foley catheters are frequently used in the anterior gastric wall and are held in place by a purse-string suture.   *(2:326)*

113. **(D)** Hemovac closed-wound suction drains are placed in radical neck dissection wounds.   *(32:654)*

114. **(B)** The Penrose drain is a thin-walled cylinder of radiopaque Latex used to maintain a vent for the escape of fluid or air from the wound.   *(2:248)*

115. **(D)** A Pezzar or mushroom catheter is for drainage of body cavities; the others are commonly used ureteral catheter tips.   *(2:354–355)*

116. **(B)** The Gibbons is an indwelling stent catheter. Stone baskets are Dormia, Johnson, Levant, and Lomac.
(2:355)

117. **(A)** The Garceau, Braasch bulb, or whistle tip may be used to dilate the ureter.   *(2:355)*

118. **(D)** The urologist visualizes the ureteral orifice through the cystoscope. The ureteral catheter is then inserted through the instrument and introduced into the ureter.
(2:354)

119. **(D)** Moisten the drain in saline before handing it to the surgeon.   *(2:248)*

120. **(C)** The cigarette drain is made of soft rubber and is used to maintain a vent for the escape of fluid. It is a Penrose drain with a gauze strip inside. It is believed that this helps prevent adhesions.   *(25:81)*

121. **(B)** T tubes come in various sizes and crossbar lengths. They are used for drainage of tubular structures, e.g., the common bile duct.   *(22:147)*

122. **(C)** The stone basket has a fine wire or nylon basket which can ensnare a calculus located in the lower third of the ureter.   *(2:355)*

123. **(D)** The CVP catheter is usually inserted by cutdown or percutaneously into the subclavian vein or one of its feeding tributaries.   *(2:190)*

124. **(A)** Blood samples should be sent to the lab immediately. If more than 10 minutes elapse between blood drawing and analysis, the analysis cannot be considered accurate. In the event of delay, the syringe with blood should be immediately immersed in ice and refrigerated at near-freezing temperature.   *(2:190)*

125. **(A)** Indwelling catheters filled with conductive fluid, probes inserted into great vessels, and electrodes implanted about the heart multiply the potential for electrocution because they can be conductors of electricity.   *(2:284)*

126. **(C)** Hegar dilators are cervical dilators. The others are all used for urethral dilation.   *(2:357)*

127. **(B)** This system is used to apply suction to a large closed-wound site postoperatively. A constant, negative vacuum evacuates tissue fluid and blood to promote healing by reducing edema and media for microbial growth.   *(2:247)*

128. **(A)** Pressure from the Foley catheter balloon inserted after closure of the urethra helps obtain hemostasis. Either 30-cc or 75-cc balloons are used for hemostasis.   *(2:360; 22:143)*

129. **(B)** Suction tubing with a Luki tube collects washing specimens during a bronchoscopy.   *(32:368)*

130. **(C)** A Gomco suction pump (mechanically, through creation of a vacuum) allows fluid to flow from one receptacle to another.   *(7:729)*

131. **(D)** A Pezzar is a self-retaining catheter, also known as a mushroom. It is used to drain the bladder suprapubically. It is occasionally used to drain the gallbladder.   *(32:188, 246)*

132. **(B)** The Miller-Abbott is a common nasogastric tube for gastrointestinal decompression. The tube has holes in several locations near the tip to permit withdrawal of contents.   *(2:246)*

133. **(C)** The third lumen provides a means for continuous irrigation of the bladder for a time postoperatively to prevent formation of clots in the bladder.   *(2:359)*

E. EQUIPMENT

134. **(C)** The image intensifier converts the x-ray beam through the body into a fluoroscopic optic image projected onto a television screen.   *(2:291)*

135. **(A)** Extracorporeal refers to the outside of the body. Many cardiac surgical procedures are done while the patient is placed on partial or complete cardiopulmonary bypass (extracorporeal circulation). A pump removes blood from the systemic circulation, filters it, passes it through an oxygenator, and returns it to the patient via a cannula in the ascending aorta or the femoral artery. The oxygenated blood is used by the organs and tissues of the body and then returned to the pump or heart-lung machine, where the process is once again repeated.   *(7:553)*

136. **(C)** The Apgar score is a system that scores an infant's physical condition 1 minute after birth. The heart rate, respiration, muscle tone, color, and stimuli response are scored. The maximum total score for a normal baby is 10. Those with low scores require immediate attention if they are to survive.   *(36:115)*

137. **(D)** An electroencephalogram (EEG) records electrical activity of the brain via electrodes applied to the scalp.   *(7:1179)*

138. **(A)** The Berman locator is a small but extremely sensitive version of a mine detector; it can indicate the exact location of a metallic foreign body.   *(2:409)*

139. **(C)** A roentgen is a unit for describing an exposure dose of radiation. It was discovered by Wilhelm Roentgen in 1895.   *(36:1502)*

140. **(D)** The inactive electrode which disperses current is incorporated in the bipolar unit forceps used by the surgeon. One side of the forcep is the active electrode, the other side is inactive. The current returns directly through the forcep to the machine.   *(2:251)*

141. **(D)** The size of the graft obtained from a Reese dermatome is limited by the width and length of the drum.   *(2:446)*

142. **(A)** After removal of the split-thickness mesh-graft with dermatome, the graft is placed on a plastic dermacarrier, upside down. The mesher then cuts small parallel slits in the graft. This permits expansion to three times its original size.   *(2:447)*

143. **(B)** The dissecting or operating microscope has a variety of magnification ranging from 6x to 40x. This is an improvement over the use of the Loupe, which magnifies 2x to 2.8x.   *(32:757)*

144. **(B)** Tourniquets are dangerous if not applied and set carefully. The proper setting for an arm is 250 to 300 mm Hg. The proper setting for a leg is 400 to 500 mm Hg. *(32:461)*

145. **(C)** The 3M minidriver is a valuable power tool because of its versatility of use. The Swanson reamer chuck, the Jacobs drill chuck, the sagittal saw chuck, and the K-wire driver are all available attachments. The mini-driver has no oscillating saw chuck. *(6:216)*

146. **(B)** Use of the Hall air-driver for drilling requires the addition of a Jacobs drill bit chuck. *(6:216)*

147. **(D)** The Ernst appliances are a set of instruments used to insert radium for cervical malignancies. *(32:329)*

148. **(C)** Phacoemulsification (the fragmentation of a lens by use of ultrasonic energy and its subsequent aspiration from the capsule) is accomplished by the use of a Cavitron unit. *(32:687)*

149. **(C)** Compressed nitrogen is the power source in all air-powered equipment. *(32:729)*

150. **(B)** After the kidneys are "harvested" from the donor, they are immediately placed in a cold saline solution, surrounded by ice, or placed on a hypothermic pulsatile perfusion machine (such as the Waters' perfusion machine) for transport. *(32:300)*

151. **(A)** The Ronjair, an air-powered rongeur used in surgery of the spine, has interchangeable attachments for Leksell, Luer, and Kerrison rongeurs. *(33:729)*

152. **(D)** Cardiac procedures are performed while the patient is placed on partial or complete cardiopulmonary bypass. The patient is placed on a machine composed of a mechanical pump that stimulates the action of the left ventricle and an oxygenator that simulates the function of the lungs. *(7:553)*

153. **(A)** The mechanical pump simulates the pumping action of the left ventricle. *(7:442)*

154. **(D)** The cerebrospinal fluid spaces in and around the brain may be seen by x-ray exam when the cerebrospinal fluid is replaced with a gas. The gas (air) serves as the contrast medium because air is less dense than fluid to roentgen rays. This is an x-ray study of the ventricles and subarachnoid space of the brain. Air is introduced via a lumbar puncture. *(7:1175)*

155. **(B)** Loupes are glasses with telescopic lenses used for magnification in microvascular surgery and nerve repair. *(32:537)*

156. **(A)** Electric current will flow to the ground or a neutral potential. Therefore, a proper channel must be provided to disperse the current released through the active electrode and provide the return from the tissues back to the electrosurgical unit. *(2:251)*

157. **(B)** Fluoroscopy through the image intensifier is the procedure of choice for inserting an endocardial lead. *(32:422)*

158. **(B)** There are two types of pacemakers. The asynchronous model has a standard pace of 72 bpm. The demand model fires only when the patient's heartbeat drops below the prescribed rate. *(32:422)*

159. **(B)** After trephination of the skull, a neuroblade with dura guard is attached to the craniotome to effect a bone flap. *(32:729)*

160. **(B)** The argon laser operates in the visible light region in the blue-green spectrum. It is easily delivered to the tissue through flexible fiberoptics and can be coupled to a microscope or hand probe. Argon laser energy is primarily absorbed in tissue by melanin and hemoglobin. *(28:390)*

CHAPTER 5

Surgical Procedures
Questions

Directions: Each of the questions or incomplete statements below is followed by four suggested answer or completions. Select the best answer in each case.

A. GENERAL SURGERY

1. The term transduodenal sphincterotomy indicates surgery of the

A. hepatic duct
B. proximal end of the common bile duct
C. distal end of the common bile duct
D. pyloric sphincter

2. A tract between two epithelium-lined surfaces, open at both ends is a

A. fissure
B. fistula
C. sinus
D. keloid

3. An ulcer of the anus is called a/an

A. fissure in ano
B. anal fistula
C. pilonidal cyst
D. anal abscess

4. During an appendectomy, a purse-string suture is placed around the appendix stump in order to

A. amputate the appendicial base
B. retract the appendix
C. tie off the appendix
D. invert the stump of the appendix

5. What type of suture would be positioned into the gallbladder before a cholecystotomy is attempted?

A. retention suture
B. purse-string suture
C. traction suture
D. mattress suture

6. A forceps used to remove stones in biliary surgery is a

A. mixter
B. Lahey gall duct
C. Potts-Smith
D. Randall

7. Gastrointestinal technique is required in all of the following procedures except

A. cholecystectomy
B. low anterior colon resection
C. appendectomy
D. excision of Meckel's diverticulum

8. A hernia occurring in Hesselback's triangle is called

A. indirect
B. spigelean
C. direct
D. femoral

9. Pathologic enlargement of the male breast is called

A. subcutaneous adenoma
B. gynecomastia
C. hypoplasia
D. cystic mastitis

10. Sutures placed in a wound to prevent wound evisceration are called

A. stent
B. fixation
C. retention
D. traction

11. Surgical enlargement of the passage between the prepylorus of the stomach and the duodenum is a

A. pyloromyotomy
B. pyloroplasty
C. Billroth I
D. Billroth II

12. A Whipple operation is surgically termed a

A. pancreatectomy
B. pancreatoduodenectomy
C. pancreatic cyst marsupilization
D. transduodenal sphincterotomy

13. A left subcostal incision indicates surgery of the

A. gallbladder
B. pancreas
C. spleen
D. common bile duct

14. A lower oblique incision is a/an

A. McBurney
B. inguinal
C. paramedian
D. midabdominal

15. Which of the following instruments would *not* be found in an esophagogastrectomy?

A. automatic stapling device
B. Potts forceps
C. Alexander periosteotome
D. Mason-Judd retractor

16. What secondary surgery might be done on a patient after removal of a breast or prostate malignancy?

A. Whipple
B. hypophysectomy
C. bilateral adrenalectomy
D. lumbar sympathectomy

17. Dilation of the ampulla of Vater is considered necessary to treat

A. hepatic duct obstruction
B. pyloric obstruction
C. cardiostenosis
D. common duct stones

18. What incision is indicated for an esophagogastrectomy?

A. left paramedian
B. upper vertical midline
C. thoracoabdominal
D. full midabdominal

19. In which incision could retention sutures be used?

A. midline
B. McBurney
C. transverse
D. thoracoabdominal

20. The invagination of proximal intestine into the lumen of distal intestine is called

A. volvulus
B. intussusception
C. pyloric stenosis
D. ileal atresia

21. The procedure for removal of the pituitary gland is a

A. Whipple procedure
B. vagotomy
C. sphincterectomy
D. hypophysectomy

22. What is the primary function of the thyroid gland?

A. calcium metabolism
B. hormone regulation
C. hormone balance
D. iodine metabolism

23. Which procedure is performed for Cushing's syndrome?

A. adrenalectomy
B. hypophysectomy
C. vagotomy
D. pancreatectomy

24. The surgical procedure performed in conjunction with a total colectomy is a/an

A. colostomy
B. cecostomy
C. ileostomy
D. jejunostomy

25. Wound protection and isolation of gastrointestinal contaminants are effectively aided by use of a/an

A. plastic ring drape
B. moistened lap pad
C. adhesive vi-drape
D. Lahey bowel bag

26. Approximation of the serosal layer of the intestines is accomplished by use of

A. continuous silk suture
B. interrupted silk suture
C. continuous chromic suture
D. interrupted chromic suture

27. All of the following statements refer to pilonidal cyst surgery *except*

A. performed with elliptical incision
B. wound frequently heals by granulation
C. probes are required on setup
D. cyst is always infected

28. Fine dissecting scissors for abdominal surgery are

A. Mayo scissors
B. Potts-Smith scissors
C. Metzenbaum scissors
D. Lahey scissors

29. Upon completion of a colon anastomosis, the defect in the _____ must be closed to prevent postoperative obstruction.

A. lesser omentum
B. greater omentum
C. pelvic fascia
D. mesentery

30. The site of a pilonidal cyst formation is the

A. rectum
B. anus
C. sacrococcyx
D. lumbar region

31. Good exposure for thyroid surgery is ensured by all of the following *except*

A. slight reverse Trendelenburg position
B. hyperextension of the neck
C. utilization of skin-stay sutures
D. firm retraction of the laryngeal nerve and surrounding structures

32. An instrument used to elevate the thyroid gland during surgical excision is a

A. Babcock
B. Lahey
C. Greene
D. Jackson

33. Place the intestinal layer in order, from inside to outside.

A. serosa, mucosa, musculature
B. mucosa, submucosa, serosa
C. serosa, musculature, mucosa
D. mucosa, serosa, musculature

34. Postoperative hemorrhage or biliary drainage is decreased by suturing the liver bed of the excised gallbladder with

A. chromic 000 suture, GI needle
B. chromic 0 suture, Mayo needle
C. silk 000 suture, GI needle
D. silk 0 suture, Ferguson needle

35. Most newborn emergency surgical anomalies occur in the

A. respiratory system
B. circulatory system
C. alimentary tract
D. skeletal system

36. Which set of terms identifies the origin of a Wilm's tumor?

A. kidney, adult
B. ovary, female
C. kidney, child
D. liver, adult

37. Surgery done to prevent phimosis in a newborn is called

A. orchiopexy
B. orchiectomy
C. circumcision
D. urethral repair

38. In gallbladder surgery the liver is covered with moist laps and retracted gently upward with a/an

A. Army-Navy
B. Hibbs
C. Hohman
D. Deaver

39. An imperforation or closure of a normal opening is called

A. hypertrophy
B. atresia
C. stenosis
D. atrophy

40. Failure of the intestines to encapsulate within the peritoneal cavity of a newborn is called

A. umbilical hernia
B. omphalocele
C. hydrocele
D. intestinal extrophy

41. A congenital malformation of the chest wall with a pronounced funnel-shaped depression is called

A. truncus anteriosis
B. pectus excavatum
C. pectus carinatum
D. costochondrial separation

42. Newborn vomiting, free of bile and projectile in nature, is indicative of

A. atresia of the esophagus
B. pyloric stenosis
C. volvulus
D. intussusception

43. Hirschsprung's disease is synonymous with

A. congenital aganglionosis
B. malrotation
C. ileal stenosis
D. Meckel's diverticulum

44. The increased metabolic rate of a surgical pediatric patient establishes the need for all of the following *except*

A. oxygen
B. caloric intake
C. blood transfusions
D. fluids

45. The instrument most commonly used to grasp the mesoappendix during an appendectomy is a

A. Kelly
B. Kocher
C. Babcock
D. Allis

46. What position is *not* used for rectal surgery?

A. dorsal recumbent
B. Sims lateral
C. jackknife
D. lithotomy

47. A choledochojejunostomy is surgically known as a

A. Fredet-Ramstedt procedure
B. Roux-Y procedure
C. Torek procedure
D. Blalock-Taussig procedure

48. Utilizing electric current to close severed vessels is called

A. cauterization
B. coagulation
C. fulguration
D. desiccation

49. A surgical procedure performed to relieve esophageal obstruction due to cardiospasm is an

A. esophagectomy
B. esophagogastrectomy
C. esophagomyotomy
D. esophagogastrostomy

50. Thrombosed vessels of the rectum are known surgically as

A. polyps
B. hemorrhoids
C. fistulas
D. anorectal tumors

51. An additional table piece that is added when the patient is placed in reverse Trendelenburg position is a/an

A. shoulder brace
B. padded footboard
C. kidney rest
D. elevating pad

52. Establishment of an opening into the gallbladder to permit drainage or remove stones is a

A. choledochotomy
B. cholecystostomy
C. cholecystotomy
D. cholecystectomy

53. All of the following are complications of a gastric ulcer *except*

A. paralytic ileus
B. perforation
C. pyloric obstruction
D. hemorrhage

54. Blunt dissection of the gallbladder from the sulcus of the liver requires the use of a

A. Metzenbaum
B. Kelly
C. tampon
D. peanut

55. Following a vein stripping procedure, legs are wrapped with elastic bandages to

A. stimulate circulation
B. prevent thrombosis
C. create a compression dressing
D. encourage venous stasis

56. A minor diagnosis liver procedure is a

A. Craig needle biopsy
B. Silverman needle biopsy
C. Dorsey cannula biopsy
D. Veress needle biopsy

57. In a crisis situation, radical amputation of a limb requiring a secondary closure is called

A. AK amputation
B. guillotine amputation
C. transmetatarsal amputation
D. BK amputation

58. All of the following statements are true of fiberoptic equipment *except*

A. it is an improved method of illumination
B. it has low light intensity
C. the light is cool
D. the light is conducted through a bundle of coated glass fibers

59. To prevent abdominal infection resulting from spillage of an inflamed gallbladder, a _____ is placed in the wall of the gallbladder before removal is attempted.

A. traction suture
B. lap pad
C. trocar
D. T tube

60. What type of suture and needle are used to repair the liver bed in a cholecystectomy?

A. fine chromic suture, fine needle
B. fine silk suture, fine needle
C. heavy chromic suture, large blunt needle
D. fine silk suture, large blunt needle

61. Dysphagia is

A. painful swallowing
B. difficult swallowing
C. deficient esophageal peristalsis
D. noisy swallowing

62. All of the following are required in preparation for hepatic surgery *except*

A. adequate preparation for blood loss
B. electrocoagulation
C. fine intestinal needles for liver suture
D. portal pressure monitors

63. A cholangiogram requires all of the following *except*

A. Bakes dilators and malleable probe
B. syringes, asepto syringes, and aspirating needles
C. gastrointestinal setup
D. contrast media, catheters, T tube

64. Which incision would require cutting through Scarpa's fascia?

A. subcostal
B. inguinal
C. phannenstiel
D. McBurney

65. Portocaval shunt is indicated for all of the following *except*

A. Laennec's cirrhosis
B. esophageal varices
C. portal hypotension
D. portal hypertension

66. Which muscle may be transected in executing an upper oblique incision?

A. internal oblique
B. pyramidal muscle
C. abdominus rectus
D. external oblique

67. An abdominal incision parallel and about 4 cm lateral to the midline is a/an

A. subcostal
B. paramedian rectus
C. transverse
D. inguinal

68. An irreducible hernia whose abdominal contents have become ischemic is called a/an

A. incarcerated hernia
B. sliding hernia
C. Spigelean hernia
D. strangulated hernia

B. GYNECOLOGIC PROCEDURES

69. The main blood supply of the female pelvis is derived from the

A. branches of the ascending aorta
B. median sacral arteries
C. common iliac arteries
D. ovarian arteries

70. Reorganization of the graafian follicles after ovulation results in formation of the

A. immature ovum
B. corpus luteum
C. cortex
D. medulla

71. The outer surfaces of the fallopian tube are covered by

A. mucosa
B. peritoneum
C. endometrium
D. myometrium

72. The external female organs are known collectively as

A. perineum
B. vagina
C. vulva
D. vestibule

73. An iodine staining of the cervix to determine abnormal cervical cell growth is called a

A. Rubin's test
B. Papanicolaou smear
C. Schiller's test
D. Rinne test

74. A procedure done on young women who evidence benign uterine tumors but who wish to preserve fertility is a

A. subtotal hysterectomy
B. Wertheim procedure
C. myomectomy
D. Le Fort procedure

75. A radical procedure involving the reproductive, gastrointestinal, genitourinary, vascular, and lymphatic systems is a

A. Wertheim procedure
B. pelvic exenteration
C. abdominal perineal resection
D. Manchester procedure

76. Radiologic investigation of the uterus and tubes is a

A. Rubin's test
B. hysterogram
C. hysterosalpingogram
D. hysteroscopy

77. Sterility can be accomplished by all of the following procedures *except*

A. laparoscopy
B. minilaparotomy
C. posterior colpotomy
D. culdoscopy

78. A scheduled procedure whose ultimate surgical goal involves abdominal, perineal, and groin dissection is a

A. radical vulvectomy and lymphadenectomy
B. Wertheim procedure
C. pelvic exenteration
D. Manchester procedure

79. All of the following self-retaining retractors are used for pelvic surgery *except*

A. Martin ring
B. Balfour
C. Wullstein
D. O'Sullivan-O'Conner

80. All of the following are uterine ligaments *except*

A. broad
B. round
C. external lateral
D. uterosacral

81. Extrauterine pregnancies can occur in the

A. abdominal cavity and tube
B. ovary and pelvic ligaments
C. abdominal cavity and corpus luteum
D. pelvic ligaments and tube

82. Benign invasion of the myometrium by endometrial tissue is called

A. endometriosis
B. adenomyosis
C. adenocarcinoma
D. malignant stromatosis

83. A Foley catheter is placed into the presurgical hysterectomy patient to

A. record accurate intake and output
B. distend the bladder during surgery
C. avoid injury to the bladder
D. maintain a dry perineum postoperatively

84. What would an anterior and posterior repair accomplish?

A. repair of cystocele and retrocele
B. repair of vesicovaginal fistula
C. repair of vesicourethral fistula
D. repair of labial hernia

85. Reconstruction of the cervical canal is called

A. cervicectomy
B. trachelorrhaphy
C. vulvectomy
D. circlage

86. An incision made during normal labor to facilitate delivery with less trauma to the mother is a/an

A. colpotomy
B. colporrhaphy
C. episiotomy
D. celiotomy

87. Cervical carcinoma-in-situ can be classified as

A. limited to the epithelial layer, noninvasive
B. microinvasive
C. clinically obvious
D. vaginal extension limitations

88. The most common cancer of the reproductive system in the female is

A. ovarian
B. endometrial
C. cervical
D. adnexal

89. Backward displacement of the uterus in the pelvic cavity is termed

A. antiversion
B. prolapse
C. retroversion
D. displacement

90. To confirm the diagnosis of ectopic pregnancy, it is sometimes necessary to perform a

A. Rubin's test
B. culdocentesis
C. paracentesis
D. laparotomy

91. Tuboplasty is

A. salpingectomy
B. salpingostomy
C. salpingogram
D. tubul insufflation

92. Large glands located on either side of the distal vagina in the labia majora are the

A. Skene's glands
B. para-urethral ducts
C. Bartholin's glands
D. Cowper's glands

93. The most commonly identified ovarian cyst is the

A. chocolate
B. follicle
C. corpus luteum
D. dermoid

94. A herniation of the cul-de-sac of Douglas is a/an

A. cystocele
B. rectocele
C. hydrocele
D. enterocele

95. A vesicourethral abdominal suspension is known as a

A. Le Fort
B. Wertheim
C. Marshall-Marchetti
D. Shirodkar

96. The most common female genital fistula is a/an

A. vesicovaginal
B. ureterovaginal
C. urethrovaginal
D. rectovaginal

97. Direct visualization of the pelvic organs through the pouch of Douglas is called

A. laparoscopy
B. hysteroscopy
C. culdoscopy
D. peritonoscopy

98. Papanicolaou indicates

A. removal of small pieces of cervix for exam

B. cytologic study of cervical smear
C. staining of the cervix for study
D. direct visualization of pelvic organs

99. The end result of nonfertilization is

A. menopause
B. menstruation
C. maturation
D. ovulation

100. All of the following are modifications of dorsal recumbent position *except*

A. Trendelenburg
B. lithotomy
C. reverse Trendelenburg
D. Kraske

101. Pressure against soft tissues of the leg in lithotomy position predisposes the patient to develop

A. muscle strain
B. radial nerve damage
C. venous thrombosis
D. capillary hemorrhage

102. Abnormal uterine bleeding at irregular intervals is

A. amenorrhea
B. menorrhagia
C. metrorrhagia
D. dystmenorrhea

103. The position used when performing a laparoscopy is

A. lithotomy
B. reverse Trendelenburg
C. supine
D. Fowler's

104. Which incision is used in laparoscopy?

A. infraumbilical
B. phannenstiel
C. lower oblique
D. infraumbilical

C. EYE, EAR, NOSE, THROAT, AND PLASTIC SURGERY

105. Dilating eye drops are called

A. mydriatics
B. miotics
C. myopics
D. oxytocics

106. A cataract lens is frequently frozen and extracted by use of a

A. Cavitron unit
B. keratome
C. cryoprobe
D. laser

107. The most preventable cause of blindness is

A. cornea scarring
B. cataract
C. retinal detachment
D. glaucoma

108. The most common cause of retinal detachment is

A. nearsightedness
B. trauma
C. aging process
D. inflammation

109. Intraocular pressure is measured with a/an

A. caliper
B. tonometer
C. ophthalmoscope
D. exophthalometer

110. Sagging and eversion of the lower lid is

A. entropion
B. blepharitis
C. ectropion
D. ptosis

111. Removal of the entire eyeball is

A. keratoplasty
B. exenteration
C. enucleation
D. evisceration

112. Mary V. is diagnosed as having open-angle glaucoma. A surgical procedure establishing an artificial method of draining aqueous fluid to reduce intraocular pressure is called

A. iridectomy
B. iridencleisis
C. scleral buckling
D. trabeculectomy

113. Removal of a portion of an ocular muscle with reattachment is called

A. recession
B. resection
C. strabismus
D. myomectomy

114. Opacity of the vitreous humor is treated by performing a

A. cataract removal
B. scleral buckling procedure
C. vitrectomy
D. goniotomy

115. Fine hooks available in varying angles are essential dissecting tools to perform a

A. myringotomy
B. tonsillectomy
C. stapedectomy
D. mastoidectomy

116. A surgical schedule would describe the procedure to treat otitis media as a

A. myringotomy
B. stapes mobilization
C. fenestration operation
D. Wullstein procedure

117. Restoration of hearing in a patient with otosclerosis is known surgically as

A. labyrinthectomy
B. mastoidectomy
C. fenestration procedure
D. stapedectomy

118. Re-establishment of a functioning linkage between the incus and the inner ear is a

A. stapedectomy
B. labyrinthectomy
C. stapes mobilization
D. myringoplasty

119. Restoration of hearing loss due to obstruction of the eustachian tube by an adjacent organ is

A. stapedectomy
B. tonsillectomy
C. labyrinthectomy
D. adenoidectomy

120. Hearing loss is measured by

A. amperes
B. pitch
C. frequencies
D. decibels

121. Untreated acute otitis media may result in

A. mastoiditis
B. adenoiditis
C. Bell's palsy
D. otosclerosis

122. A cosmetic procedure done to correct protruding ears is called a

A. stapes mobilization
B. tympanoplasty
C. blepharoplasty
D. otoplasty

123. All of the following organs are responsible for equilibrium *except* the

A. semicircular canals
B. utricle
C. cochlea
D. saccule

124. A term referring to the ear is

A. aura
B. oral
C. aural
D. auric

125. In the physiology of hearing, sound waves collect in the _____, and pass on to hit the _____.

A. auricle, ossicles
B. external canal, internal canal
C. auricle, tympanic membrane
D. ossicles, oval window

126. Removal of tissue at the roof of the nasopharynx and behind the posterior choanae to facilitate breathing and prevent recurrent attacks of otitis media is

A. adenoidectomy
B. tonsillectomy
C. turbinectomy
D. polypectomy

127. All of the following are required for repair of a nasal fracture *except*

A. bayonet forceps
B. Ballinger swivel knife
C. splint
D. speculum

128. Surgical correction of a deviated septum is known as a/an

A. antrostomy
B. submucous resection
C. rhinoplasty
D. turbinectomy

129. A term referring to nosebleed is

A. sinusitis
B. rhinitis
C. epistaxis
D. rhinorrhea

130. The correct instrument in a rhinoplasty to remove the septal cartilage and deformity would be

A. Kerrison forceps
B. Jansen-Middleton forceps
C. McCoy forceps
D. Myles curette

131. A suprasternal notch incision is indicative of a

A. tracheostomy
B. thoacoplasty
C. mediastinoscopy
D. cardiac surgery

132. All of the following instruments can be found on a nasal setup *except*

A. Freer elevator
B. bayonet forceps
C. Potts forceps
D. Frazier suction tube

133. Which of the following medications would be used as a topical anesthetic prior to nasal surgery?

A. Numorphan
B. codeine
C. cocaine
D. Xylocaine

134. The nasal sinus located between the nose and the orbits is the

A. frontal
B. sphenoid
C. ethmoid
D. maxillary

135. To establish a tracheostomy, a midline incision is created in the neck, below the _____.

A. suprasternal notch
B. hyoid bone
C. cricoid cartilage
D. corniculate cartilage

136. The only portion of a tracheostomy tube that may be removed and cleansed is the

A. sheath
B. inner cannula
C. outer cannula
D. stylette

137. Excision of the laryngeal structures above the true vocal cords is a

A. supraglottic laryngectomy
B. total laryngectomy
C. radical neck dissection
D. laryngofissurectomy

138. The majority of benign salivary gland tumors occur in the gland _____.

A. sublingual
B. submaxillary
C. parotid
D. submandibular

139. The purpose for performing a dacrocysto-rhinostomy is to

A. correct a nasal defect
B. create openings in the maxillary sinus
C. correct ectropian
D. create an opening for tear flow

140. What is otosclerosis?

A. formation of spongy bone in the ear
B. ringing in the ears
C. hardening of the tympanic membrane
D. infection in the ear

141. Which position is chosen for the adult patient undergoing a local tonsillectomy?

A. Sims
B. semi-Fowler's
C. dorsal recumbent
D. Trendelenburg

142. All of the following can be found on a tonsillectomy setup *except*

A. Yankauer suction
B. Hurd dissector
C. pillar retractor
D. Cottle cartilage holder

143. What mode would be utilized to maintain drainage postoperatively in radical neck surgery?

A. Penrose drain
B. Hemovac
C. sump drain
D. T tube

144. Glossectomy indicates removal of the

A. tongue
B. lips
C. mandible
D. gum tissue

145. A graft containing epidermis and only a portion of the dermis is called a

A. split thickness graft
B. full thickness Wolfe graft
C. composite graft
D. full thickness pinch graft

146. A progressive disease of the palmar fascia is termed

A. Dupuytren's contracture
B. tendonitis
C. carpal tunnel syndrome
D. synovitis

147. The amount of pressure used to inflate a tourniquet depends on all of the following *except*

A. patient's age
B. size of extremity
C. depth of surgical incision
D. systolic blood pressure

148. A rubber bandage used to exsanguinate a limb previous to inflation of a tourniquet is called a/an

A. Kling bandage
B. Esmarch bandage
C. Kerlex gauze
D. Elastoplast wrap

149. Microtia refers to

A. protrusion of the external ear
B. absence of the external ear
C. abnormally small ears
D. premature closing of cranial sutures

150. All of the following are dermatomes *except*

A. Reese
B. Padgett-Hood
C. Stryker
D. Brown

151. Which of the following is considered a disadvantage when using a silicone implant?

A. minimal tissue reaction
B. lack of alteration by the body
C. stability in heat and time
D. adherence to tissue

152. A flap that is moved from one part of the body to another with a stalk attached to the donor site is called a

A. direct flap
B. pedicle flap
C. free flap
D. composite flap

153. Most fractures of the body of the mandible are immobilized by use of

A. open reduction with arch bars
B. closed reduction with arch bars
C. open reduction with stainless steel wiring
D. closed reduction with stainless steel wiring

154. The surgical procedure indicated to correct prognathism or micrognathia is

A. blepharoplasty
B. rhinoplasty
C. mentoplasty
D. otoplasty

155. What position is a patient placed in following a T&A?

A. on side, horizontally
B. on stomach, head lowered
C. on back, sitting up straight
D. on back, head lowered

156. Which procedure requires the use of a wooden tongue depressor?

A. radical neck
B. tonsillectomy
C. split thickness graft
D. vocal cord polypectomy

D. GENITOURINARY PROCEDURES

157. Nonmalignant enlargement of the prostate is termed

A. prostatitis
B. BPH
C. balanitis
D. prostatism

158. Large urethral strictures in the male can be dilated by the use of a

A. filiform catheter
B. Van Buren sound
C. Phillips catheter
D. coudé catheter

159. A staghorn stone is one that lodges and continues to grow, eventually filling the

A. renal calyx
B. space of Retzius
C. ureter
D. hilum

160. Carcinoma of the prostate or breast frequently requires removal of the _____ glands to diminish _____ secretion.

A. adrenal, adrenaline
B. adrenal, enzyme
C. adrenal, steroid
D. adrenal, hormone

161. Which of the following is *not* considered a permanent urinary diversion?

A. ileal conduit

B. ureterosigmoidostomy
C. cutaneous ureterostomy
D. nephrostomy

162. Rib removal for surgical exposure of the kidney requires all of the following *except* a/an

A. Alexander periosteotome
B. Doyen raspatory
C. Heaney clamp
D. Bethune

163. A surgical procedure done to correct the abnormality in which the urethral meatus is situated on the upper side of the penis is called

A. urethral meatotomy
B. epispadias repair
C. hypospadias repair
D. urethroplasty

164. Removal of a testis or the testes is called

A. orchiopexy
B. orchiectomy
C. epididymectomy
D. vasectomy

165. All of the following are incisional options in a nephrectomy *except*

A. simple flank
B. thoracoabdominal
C. Kocher's
D. retroperitoneal

166. Temporary diversion of urinary drainage by means of an external catheter which drains the kidney pelvis is called

A. vesicostomy
B. nephrostomy
C. pyelostomy
D. cystostomy

167. All of the following are components of a resectoscope *except* a/an

A. sheath
B. obturator
C. lithotrite
D. working element

168. Conductive lubricants must *never* be used on the sheath of a resectoscope because it

A. restricts ease of introduction
B. provides a path for electrical current
C. encourages nosocomial infections
D. obstructs the visual ability of the surgeon

169. All of the following are types of cystoscopes *except*

A. Brown-Buerger
B. Stern-McCarthy
C. McCarthy
D. Wappler

170. Microscopic reversal of the male sterilization procedure is termed

A. spermatogenesis
B. orchiopexy
C. vasovasostomy
D. vasovasotomy

171. Surgically created arteriovenous fistulas of the forearm form an anastomosis between the,

A. brachial artery and the cephalic vein
B. radial artery and the cephalic vein
C. radial artery and the basilic vein
D. brachial artery and the basilic vein

172. Which muscles are divided when approaching the kidney through a lumbar approach?

A. superior rectus
B. peroneus tertius
C. platysma
D. internal and external oblique

173. To "harvest a kidney" is a phrase denoting a _____ kidney.

A. pyogenic
B. nonfunctioning
C. cadaver's
D. dropped

174. The process of removing waste products from the blood of a patient in renal failure is called

A. filtration
B. revascularization
C. perfusion
D. hemodialysis

175. Continuous irrigation following a transurethral resection of the prostate is accomplished by use of a

A. suprapubic cystotomy tube
B. 30-cc 3-way Foley catheter
C. 5-cc 3-way Foley catheter
D. 30-cc 2-way Foley catheter

176. Which surgical procedure is indicated for removal of a benign, grossly hypertrophied prostate?

A. retropubic prostatectomy
B. transurethral prostatectomy
C. perineal prostatectomy
D. suprapubic prostatectomy

177. When the prostate gland is removed through an abdominal incision into the prostate capsule it is called a _____ prostatectomy.

A. perineal
B. suprapubic
C. retropubic
D. transurethral

178. A renal disease process generally regarded as secondary to renal hypertension is

A. glomerulonephritis
B. nephrosclerosis
C. nephrosis
D. hydronephrosis

179. Disease in the pelvis of the kidney is termed

A. nephritis
B. pyelonephrosis
C. urethritis
D. cystostomosis

180. Abdominal surgery for removal of stones from a kidney is called

A. pyelolithotomy
B. nephrolithotomy
C. litholapaxy
D. pyelotomy

181. Orchiopexy can be defined as

A. fixation of an ovary
B. uterine suspension
C. testicle removal
D. fixation of a testicle

182. Abdominal resection of the prostate gland through an incision into the bladder is known surgically as a

A. retropubic prostatectomy
B. suprapubic prostatectomy
C. transurethral prostatectomy
D. suprapubic cystostomy

183. A postoperative complication associated with prostatectomy is

A. orchitis
B. balanitis
C. epididymitis
D. urethritis

184. Seminal fluid is manufactured mostly in the seminal vesicles and the

A. epididymis
B. tunica vaginalis
C. Cowper's gland
D. prostate gland

185. Prolonged torsion of the spermatic cord can lead to

A. loss of testicle
B. epididymitis
C. scrotal hernia
D. acute orchitis

186. Hydroureter refers to

A. excessive secretion of urine
B. edema or cyst of the ovary
C. a sac or bursa containing fluid
D. distention of the ureter with fluid

187. The irrigating solution most commonly used during transurethral surgery is

A. saline
B. water
C. glycine
D. physiosol

188. Urethritis has caused meatal stenosis in a male. The surgical correction of this condition is

A. frenulotomy
B. meatotomy
C. urethral dilation
D. extirpation of the penis

189. Hydroelectronic fragmentation of calculi transurethrally is called

A. litholapaxy
B. lithopexy
C. lithotripsy
D. cystolithotomy

190. A pigtail ureteral stent accomplishes which of the following goals?

A. palliative upper urinary tract diversion
B. ureteral bypass
C. ease of stone removal
D. dilation of urethral stricture

191. Circumcision refers to

A. removal of the foreskin
B. removal of the glans
C. widening of the urethral opening
D. lengthening of the foreskin

E. THORACIC, CARDIOVASCULAR, AND PERIPHERAL VASCULAR PROCEDURES

192. All of the following statements are true of thoraseal disposable Pleuravacs *except*

A. closely resemble the three-bottle drainage unit
B. air inlet must be sealed to prevent contamination
C. must be replaced when full, not emptied
D. raising above level of bedside is contraindicated

193. Passage of a sterile catheter into the heart via the brachial or femoral artery for the purpose of image intensification is called

A. angiography
B. arteriography
C. cardiac catheterization
D. cardioscopy

194. One of the most common complications following a median sternotomy is

A. deformity
B. atelectasis
C. bronchiopleural fistula
D. brachial plexus injury

195. Removal of air or blood from the pleural cavity by means of needle aspiration is

A. internal stabilization
B. paracentesis
C. thoracentesis
D. pneumothorax

196. What incision is utilized to surgically remove scalene nodes for biopsy?

A. axillary approach
B. cervical mediastinotomy
C. supraclavicular approach
D. transsternal bilateral thoracotomy

197. A reduction of negative pressure on one side of the thoracic cavity which causes the negative pressure on the normal side to pull in an effort to equalize pressure is called

A. vital capacity
B. mediastinal shift
C. subatmospheric pressure
D. pneumothorax

198. Surgical removal of fibrinous deposits on the visceral and parietal pleura is called

A. posteriolateral thoracoplasty
B. talc poudrage
C. decortication of the lung
D. anterior thoracoplasty

199. When a rib is removed the remaining bone edges are trimmed with a

A. Stille-Leur rongeur
B. Doyen raspatory
C. Bethune shear
D. Lebsche knife

200. A wedge resection of lung is most easily accomplished by the use of a/an

A. TA 90 staple unit
B. TA 55 staple unit
C. EEA staple unit
D. LDS staple unit

201. Which forceps would be used to grasp and immobilize the lung during a lobectomy or pneumonectomy?

A. Rummel
B. Walton
C. Lovelace
D. Willauer-Allis

202. The shunt between the aorta and the pulmonary artery which exists prenatally but closes soon after birth is called

A. pulmonary artery bonding
B. patent ductus arteriosis
C. tricuspid valve
D. coarctation of the aorta

203. Which of the following instruments would *not* be found on a cardiothoracic setup?

A. Satinsky clamp
B. Rumel tourniquet
C. Allen clamp
D. Potts scissors

204. All of the following materials are used for cardiac prosthesis *except*

A. Dacron
B. silicone rubber
C. porcine heterografts
D. nylon

205. All of the following are components of a cardiopulmonary bypass system *except*

A. oxygenator
B. heat exchanger
C. ventricular fibrillator
D. pump

206. The term used to denote the function accomplished by the cardiopulmonary bypass machine is

A. diversion
B. dialysis
C. perfusion
D. profusion

207. Plaque removal from a vessel is termed

A. embolectomy
B. thrombectomy
C. shunt
D. endarterectomy

208. The most frequent condition requiring the use of a permanent pacemaker is

A. coronary insufficiency
B. mitral insufficiency
C. heart block
D. aortic valvular stenosis

209. A transvenous insertion of a pacemaker electrode goes via the external jugular or the cephalic vein and is passed by way of the superior vena cava into the

A. left atrium
B. right ventricle
C. sinoatrial node
D. right atrium

210. Which of the following would *not* appear on a pacemaker transvenous insertion setup?

A. Potts scissors
B. #11 knife blade
C. peripheral vascular clamps
D. tunneling instrument

211. Pacemakers may be powered by all of the following methods *except*

A. mercury-zinc
B. lithium iodide
C. nickel-zinc
D. nuclear energy

212. The most common congenital cardiac anomaly in the cyanotic group is

A. tricuspid atresia
B. tetralogy of Fallot
C. atrial septal defect
D. mitral stenosis

213. Intrathoracic pacemaker electrodes inserted through an extrapleural parasternal approach are referred to as

A. endocardial
B. myocardial
C. pericardial
D. epicardial

214. Decompression of the portal circulation can be achieved by all of the following *except*

A. splenorenal shunt
B. portocaval shunt
C. hepatocaval shunt
D. mesocaval shunt

215. The pathophysiologic response to varicosities is

A. ulceration
B. gangrene
C. peripheral vascular occlusion
D. venous stasis

216. Which piece of equipment would be placed on an embolectomy setup for the purpose of removing clots through an arteriotomy?

A. Wishard
B. Swanz-Ganz
C. Fogarty
D. Garceau

217. Migrating clots which have formed in the lower extremities can be intercepted on the way to the heart or lungs by a

A. Mobbin-Uddin umbrella
B. Pudenz shunt
C. Scribner shunt
D. Le Veen shunt

218. A small, springlike vascular clamp used for occluding peripheral vessels is a

A. Debakey
B. Jackson
C. Potts
D. bulldog

219. Clipping of the inferior vena cava for recurrent emboli is effected by the use of a

A. Cushing
B. Heifitz
C. Raney
D. Miles

220. Placement of a vascular graft proximal to and inclusive of the common iliac vessels will necessitate the use of a/an

A. autogenous graft
B. straight Teflon graft
C. bifurcated graft
D. polytetrafluorethylene graft

221. The ability of an arteriole to locate new passageways of distribution when peripheral occlusive disease is present is called

A. collateral circulation
B. systemic circulation
C. arterial bypass
D. referred circulation

222. Surgery performed to relieve claudication due to peripheral vascular disease is termed

A. neurotomy

B. sclerotherapy
C. fasciotomy
D. sympathectomy

223. Retraction of fine structures during vascular surgery is accomplished by use of

A. Senn's retractor
B. Penrose drain
C. malleable ribbon retractor
D. vessel loops

F. ORTHOPEDICS, PLASTER

224. A hemostatic agent capable of controlling bleeding in bone is

A. heparin
B. avitene
C. collastat
D. bone wax

225. Congenital webbing of fingers or toes is termed

A. syndactylism
B. microtia
C. choanal atresia
D. truncus arteriosis

226. A meniscectomy setup would include all of the following *except*

A. Lane bone-holding forceps
B. Blount retractors
C. Smilie knives
D. Grover meniscotome

227. A cast applied from the hips to the head which is used to immobilize cervical fractures is a

A. Minerva jacket
B. body jacket
C. shoulder spica
D. plaster shell

228. Which of the following supplies is *not* used for cast padding?

A. Webril
B. sheet wadding
C. Esmarch bandage
D. stockingette

229. A nonsurgical treatment for clavicular fracture includes immobilization by utilizing a

A. Velpeau bandage
B. figure-eight splint
C. Minerva jacket
D. shoulder spica

230. A variation of bunionectomy, in which the surgeon includes resection of the proximal third of the phalynx and possible silicone implant is called a

A. McBride procedure
B. Keller arthroplasy
C. Bankart procedure
D. metatarsal osteotomy

231. Baker's cysts are found in the

A. popliteal fossa
B. interdigital fossa
C. intercarpal joints
D. olecranon fossa

232. Benign outpouchings of synovium from intercarpal joints are called

A. ganglia
B. exostosis
C. polyps
D. synovitis

233. Compression of the median nerve at the volar surface of the wrist is known as

A. Dupuytren's contracture
B. carpal tunnel syndrome
C. ganglia
D. Volkmann's contracture

234. Chronic dislocation of the patella may predispose the patient to a condition called

A. synovitis
B. chondromalacia
C. osteoarthritis
D. osteoporosis

235. A tear in the lateral or medial knee cartilage is repaired by performing a/an

A. synovectomy
B. meniscectomy
C. patellectomy
D. arthrodesis

236. Improper seating of the head of the femur within the acetabulum requires a surgical procedure identified as a

A. hip reconstruction
B. Schneider nailing
C. derotational osteotomy
D. hip arthroplasty

237. A dorsal angulated fracture of the distal radium is commonly called a/an

A. Pott's fracture
B. os calcis
C. olecranon fracture
D. Colle's fracture

238. A fracture similar to an oblique, differing only in the length of the fracture line, is called

A. pathologic
B. comminuted
C. spiral
D. transverse

239. Nonunion of a femoral neck fracture may necessitate the use of a femoral head prosthesis implant such as a/an

A. Charnley-Miller
B. Charnley
C. McKee-Farrar
D. Austin-Moore

240. Which of the following conditions indicates a need for total hip replacement?

A. chronic hip displacement
B. rheumatoid arthritis
C. slipped epiphysis
D. transcervical fracture

241. A basic bone set includes all of the following *except*

A. mallet and chisels
B. periosteal elevators and osteotomes
C. rongeurs and gouges
D. drivers and extractors

242. A flexion deformity at the proximal joint of the four lateral toes is called

A. valgus
B. exostosis
C. hammer-toe
D. bunion

243. Joint reconstruction is known as

A. arthrodesis
B. arthroplasty
C. arthrotomy
D. arthropexy

244. Which of the following pieces of hardware is inappropriate to repair an intermedullary fracture of an adult femur?

A. Smith-Petersen nail
B. Küntscher nail
C. Schneider nail
D. Lotte's nail

245. All of the following are vital to removal of the femoral head in a total hip replacement *except*

A. Stille-Leur rongeur
B. Gigli saw
C. osteotomes
D. Mira reamer

246. An acute infection that spreads to the bone via the bloodstream is called

A. osteomalacia
B. osteomyelitis
C. osteitis
D. osteoporosis

247. A surgical procedure designed to stiffen or fuse a joint is called

A. arthropexy
B. arthroplasty
C. joint fixation
D. arthrodesis

248. A lateral curvature of the spine is

A. kyphosis
B. scoliosis
C. lordosis
D. orthosis

249. Nonsurgical treatment of scoliosis is effected by use of all the following *except*

A. Minerva jacket
B. Milwaukee brace
C. Sayre sling
D. Risser jacket

250. Polypropylene web wrap, used to immobilize fractures in lightweight casts, is cured by use of a

A. sunlamp
B. black light
C. heating lamp
D. cast dryer

251. The congenital deformity known as clubfoot is surgically referred to as

A. talipes valgus
B. talipes varus
C. hallux valgus
D. exostosis

252. In its acute stage, tuberculous arthritis produces

A. rice bodies
B. acute inflammatory abscesses
C. cold abscesses
D. joint scarring

253. Dead bone due to osteomyelitis is called

A. osteoporosis
B. necrosis
C. sequestrum
D. involucrum

254. Bone-forming cells necessary for the callus formation in fracture repair are called

A. osteoid
B. osteoblasts
C. ossification
D. fibroblasts

255. Increased porosity of bone is referred to as

A. osteoporosis
B. osteomyelitis
C. ossification
D. ecchymosis

256. Place the stages of fracture healing in their correct order: (1) hematoma, (2) callus ossification, (3) cellular proliferation, (4) callus formation, (5) consolidation

A. 1,2,5,4,3
B. 1,3,2,4,5
C. 1,3,4,2,5
D. 1,4,3,2,5

257. The most common of all joint diseases is the degeneration of articular cartilage in the joints. This condition is known as

A. rheumatoid arthritis
B. osteoarthritis
C. osteoporosis
D. ankylosing spondylitis

258. Surgical intervention (with resultant fusion) to alleviate deformity of ankylosing spondylitis is called a/an

A. modified wedge osteotomy
B. derotational osteotomy
C. innominate osteotomy
D. laminectomy

259. A malignant disease of plasma cells that infiltrates bone and soft tissue is known as

A. giant cell tumor
B. multiple myeloma
C. osteogenic sarcoma
D. Paget's disease

260. Adult rickets is known as

A. osteoporosis
B. chondromalacia
C. osteomalacia
D. osteitis deformans

261. When Harrington rods are inserted, it is imperative to have a set of _____ on the surgical table.

A. lag screws
B. hex nuts
C. malleolus screws
D. compression screws

262. To insert a Küntscher nail, all of the following are needed *except*

A. Hudson brace and reamer
B. femur guide pin
C. Bennett retractors
D. awl reamer

263. Which of the following instruments would *not* be found in a lumbar laminectomy?

A. Kerrison rongeur
B. Taylor retractor
C. Cushing rongeur
D. Cobb elevators

264. Plaster is ready for application

A. when air bubbles cease to rise
B. when air bubbles begin to rise
C. after 2 minutes of submersion
D. after 10 minutes of submersion

265. Which fracture most commonly occurs in childhood?

A. spiral
B. compound
C. greenstick
D. comminuted

G. NEUROSURGERY

266. Michele clips are

A. skin clips
B. hemostatic clips
C. aneurysm clips
D. hemostatic scalp clips

267. What surgical procedure requires postsurgical application of Crutchfield tongs?

A. cervical laminectomy
B. cervical decompression
C. cervical rhizotomy
D. percutaneous cervical cordotomy

268. A surgical procedure used most frequently to control intractable pain of terminal cancer is called a

A. sympathectomy
B. neurectomy
C. cordotomy
D. thermocoagulation

269. A neurologic study in which radiopaque substance is injected into the subarachnoid space through a lumbar puncture is called a/an

A. cerebral angiography
B. myelogram
C. encephalogram
D. diskogram

270. Increased intracranial pressure due to tumors, head surgery, or cerebral vascular accidents results in all of the following symptoms *except*

A. vomiting
B. reduced responsiveness
C. changed vital signs
D. equal pupil response

271. The most common cause of intracerebral hemorrhage is

A. congenital A-V malformation
B. congenital aneurysm
C. hypertension
D. transient ischemic attacks

272. The contractions of involuntary muscles are controlled by the

A. sympathetic nervous system
B. autonomic nervous system
C. parasympathetic nervous system
D. central nervous system

273. A tumor arising from the covering of the brain is a/an

A. hemangioblastoma
B. angioma
C. meningioma
D. glioma

274. The recognized father of modern neurosurgery is

A. Sir Charles Sherrington
B. Harvey Cushing
C. Sir Victor Hershey
D. Sir Rickman Goodlee

275. A large, encapsulated collection of blood over one or both cerebral hemispheres which produces intracranial pressure is known as a/an

A. epidural hematoma
B. intracerebral hematoma
C. subdural hematoma
D. subarachnoid hematoma

276. A surgical procedure in which a nerve is freed from binding adhesion for relief of pain and restoration of function is termed a

A. neurexeresis
B. neurorrhaphy
C. neurotomy
D. neurolysis

277. Surgical creation of a lesion in the treatment of a disease such as Parkinson's is called

A. cryosurgery
B. diathermy
C. rhizotomy
D. pallidotomy

278. Posterior fossa exploration and exposure of the foramen magnum is executed through a

A. frontal approach
B. frontotemporal approach
C. subtemporal approach
D. suboccipital approach

279. The surgical indication represented by incomplete closure of the vertebral arches in newborns is

A. hydrocephalus
B. encephalocele
C. spina bifida
D. myelomeningocele

280. All of the following are used for hemostasis in a neurosurgical procedure *except*

A. bone wax
B. compressed cotton strips
C. bipolar coagulation
D. monopolar coagulation

281. All of the following are permanent aneurysm clips *except*

A. Scoville
B. Schwartz
C. Heifitz
D. Yasargil

282. Which of the following instruments would effect a carotid artery ligation?

A. Schwartz
B. Kerr clip
C. Selverstone clamp
D. Olivecrona clip

283. Removal of an anterior cervical disk with accompanying spinal fusion is termed a

A. Schwartz procedure
B. Cloward procedure
C. Torkildsen operation
D. stereotactic procedure

284. The condition involving premature closure of infant cranial suture lines is referred to as

A. cranioplasty
B. stereotactic surgery
C. craniosynostosis
D. transsphenoidal hypophysectomy

285. Scalp clips that are used to adhere the scalp to the bone flap during a craniotomy are called

A. McKenzie
B. Heifitz
C. Raney
D. Cushing

286. Maintenance of acceptable blood pressure and prevention of the development of air emboli in the neurosurgical patient can be effected by preoperative utilization of

A. an antigravity suit
B. Ace bandages
C. TED stockings
D. adequate body support

287. Surgical trauma to the first and second cranial nerves would cause loss of the senses of

A. smell and sight
B. smell and hearing
C. taste and sight
D. smell and taste

288. In which procedure would a Gigli saw be used?

A. laminectomy
B. Cloward procedure
C. craniotomy
D. cranioplasty

Answers and Explanations

A. GENERAL SURGERY

1. **(C)** The distal end of the common bile duct is called the sphincter of Oddi and is located where the duct enters the duodenum. A transduodenal sphincter-otomy is done to treat recurrent attacks of pancrea-titis, for it is at this junction that the pancreatic duct enters and can be obstructed due to obstruction of the common bile duct. *(32:194)*

2. **(B)** A sinus contains one open end, while a fissure is merely a crack or break in the tissue of a smooth surface. Keloids form due to an alteration in the metabolism of collagen during the fibroplastic stage of healing. *(19:346)*

3. **(A)** A benign ulcerative lesion of the anal canal is a fissure in ano. The anus must be dilated and the dis-eased tissue excised. *(2:331)*

4. **(D)** A purse-string is a continuous suture placed around the lumen of the appendicial stump to invert it. It is tightened, draw string fashion to close the lumen. *(2:262, 328)*

5. **(B)** In a cholecystotomy the fundus of the gallbladder is grasped and the proposed opening for the chole-cystotomy is encircled by means of a purse-string suture. *(32:188)*

6. **(D)** Randall stone forceps are available in various angles and are used to remove stones from inaccessible areas. *(32:186–189)*

7. **(A)** Whenever a portion of the gastrointestinal tract is entered, gastrointestinal technique must be carried out. Any instrument used after the lumen of the stomach or intestines has been entered cannot be used after it is closed. A cholecystectomy does not enter the gastrointestinal tract. *(32:210)*

8. **(C)** Hesselback's triangle is formed by the boundaries of the deep epigastric vessels laterally, the inguinal ligament inferiorly, and the abdominus rectus muscle medially. Hernias occurring here are direct. *(32:153)*

9. **(B)** Gynecomastia is a relatively common pathologic lesion that consists of bilateral or unilateral enlarge-ment of the male breast. Surgery consists of removal of all subareolar fibroglandular tissue and surgical reconstruction of the resultant defect. *(32:168)*

10. **(C)** Retention sutures may be used as a precautionary measure to prevent wound disruption and possible evisceration of the wound. *(2:263)*

11. **(B)** Pyloroplasty is the formation of a larger passage between the pylorus of the stomach and the duodenum. It may include the removal of a peptic ulcer if one is present. *(32:216)*

12. **(B)** A Whipple operation is a radical surgical excision of the head of the pancreas, the entire duodenum, a portion of the jejunum, the distal third of the stomach, and the lower half of the common bile duct. There is then re-establishment of continuity of the biliary, pancreatic, and gastrointestinal systems. This is done for carcinoma of the head of the pancreas and is a hazardous procedure. *(32:194)*

13. **(C)** A left subcostal incision is generally used for spleen surgery. The right subcostal is used for gall-bladder, common bile duct, and pancreatic surgery. *(32:204)*

14. **(B)** A lower oblique incision, either right or left, is an inguinal incision. This incision gives access to the inguinal canal and cord structures. *(2:320)*

15. **(D)** A Mason-Judd bladder retractor is used for genitourinary surgery. All of the others are intestinal or chest instruments which complete the setup for an esophagogastrectomy. *(32:275)*

16. **(C)** Certain malignancies are dependent on hormones excreted by the adrenals. Bilateral adrenalectomy may control recurrence of the malignancy. *(7:874)*

17. **(D)** After the proximal portion of the common bile duct is explored for stones, a probe and dilator are next passed through the ampulla of Vater in an attempt to release stones possibly lodged there. If this is unsuccessful, a duodenotomy must then be done to remove the stones. *(30:530)*

18. **(C)** The diseased portion of the esophagus and stomach are removed through a left thoracoabdominal incision, including a resection of the seventh, eighth, or ninth ribs. Here an anastomosis is accomplished between the disease-free ends of the stomach and the esophagus. *(32:212)*

19. **(A)** Retention or tension sutures may be used in a paramedian rectus or a vertical midline incision to ensure strength of closure. *(32:148)*

20. **(B)** The proximal intestine may be intussuscepted for many centimeters. The functional alteration results in mechanical intestinal obstruction. *(7:789)*

21. **(D)** Hypophysectomy, removal of the pituitary gland, may be done to remove primary tumors of the pituitary gland, halt the progress of hemorrhagic retinopathy, and avoid blindness due to diabetes. *(7:885)*

22. **(D)** The primary function of the thyroid gland is iodine metabolism. Injected iodides are converted into thyroid hormones for metabolism. *(32:175)*

23. **(A)** Adrenalectomy is performed for Cushing's syndrome, for adrenal tumors, and for malignancies of the breast and prostate gland. *(7:874)*

24. **(C)** The proximal end of the transected ileum is externalized through the abdominal wall. The liquid stool is collected in an ileostomy bag. Special postoperative skin care is necessary to prevent excoriation due to enzymes in the liquid stool. *(2:327)*

25. **(A)** The method of choice to effect ample wound edge protection is use of a plastic wound protector or ring drape. It is a soft, pliable, vinyl film with a circular fenestrated center. The ring protects wound edges, aids in retraction, minimizes tissue trauma, and helps keep wound edges moist. *(11:199)*

26. **(B)** After the mucosal layer of the intestines is closed with chromic suture, the outer serosal layer is closed with an interrupted suture layer of nonabsorbable material, e.g., 4-0 silk. *(11:181)*

27. **(D)** Pilonidal cysts occasionally block and become infected pilonidal abscesses. Only then are they considered septic or infected. *(32:235)*

28. **(C)** Metzenbaum scissors are fine dissection scissors used for sharp dissection of tissue in the abdomen. *(32:189)*

29. **(D)** As the anastomosis is completed the defect in the mesentery and posterior peritoneum are closed with interrupted silk sutures. *(32:231)*

30. **(C)** A pilonidal cyst is a painful, draining cyst with a fistulous tract(s) which can occur in soft tissues of the sacrococcygeal region. *(2:330)*

31. **(D)** The laryngeal nerve must be carefully identified and preserved. No pressure can be placed as it is easily damaged. *(32:177)*

32. **(B)** A Lahey vulsellum forceps is used to grasp and elevate the thyroid lobe so that sharp dissection of the lobe away from the trachea can be accomplished. *(32:177)*

33. **(B)** The layers of the large intestine from inside to outside are: mucosa, submucosa, and serosa. Mucosa suture closure is most frequently absorbable suture while the serosa layer is closed with nonabsorbable silk. *(38:621)*

34. **(A)** A remnant of 1 to 2 cm of peritoneal reflection is approximated over the gallbladder liver bed with chromic suture on a gastrointestinal needle. This step decreases chances of hemorrhage or biliary drainage. *(11:235)*

35. **(C)** Alimentary tract obstruction is the most frequent cause of emergency surgery in the newborn. The most common sites are in the esophagus, duodenum, ileum, colon, and anus. *(2:462)*

36. **(C)** Nephrectomy is necessary to resect a Wilm's tumor, a sarcoma of the kidney that develops rapidly in children usually under 5 years of age. *(2:463)*

37. **(C)** Excision of the foreskin of the penis may be done to prevent phimosis (in which the foreskin becomes tightly wrapped around the tip of the glans penis) or to remove redundant foreskin. *(2:463)*

38. **(D)** A Deaver or Harrington retractor is used to gently retract the liver during gallbladder surgery. Its width prevents damage to the liver when padded with moist laps. *(17:228)*

39. **(B)** Atresia is an imperforation or closure of an opening. Atresia and stenosis (a narrowing of an opening) are the most common causes of obstruction in a newborn.
(2:462)

40. **(B)** Failure of the intestines to become encapsulated within the peritoneal cavity during fetal development results in herniation through a midline defect in the abdominal wall at the umbilicus. This is termed an omphalocele.
(2:463)

41. **(B)** A congenital malformation of the chest wall, pectus excavatum, is characterized by a pronounced funnel-shaped depression over the lower end of the sternum.
(2:467)

42. **(B)** The first sign of pyloric stenosis is projectile vomiting free of bile. The surgical procedure for repair is a pyloromyotomy. The muscles of the pylorus are incised to relieve the stenosis.
(32:791)

43. **(A)** Hirschprung's disease is characterized by the presence of a segment of colon that lacks ganglia (congenital aganglionosis). Surgery for this anomaly requires several biopsies to locate the section of bowel with normal ganglia, followed by resection of that portion which is aganglionic.
(32:793)

44. **(C)** Due to the increased demands of surgical stress, oxygen, calories, and fluids must be increased. Blood is not given unless there is a need.
(32:780)

45. **(C)** After the abdomen is opened through a McBurney's incision, the mesoappendix is grasped with a Babcock and the appendix is gently dissected away from the cecum.
(32:294)

46. **(A)** Dorsal recumbent position is synonymous with supine and not practical for rectal surgery. Sims lateral (knee-chest), jackknife (Kraske), and lithotomy may all be used.
(32:232)

47. **(B)** The Roux-Y procedure re-establishes the flow of bile into the biliary tract by anastomosing the stump of the common bile duct into the jejunum. This procedure is usually performed to bypass an obstructing lesion of the biliary tract.
(14:109)

48. **(B)** The use of electric current for the purpose of closing severed vessels is called coagulation.
(14:57)

49. **(C)** This myotomy of the esophagogastric junction relieves the stricture and allows food to pass unrestricted into the stomach.
(32:216)

50. **(B)** Varicosities of veins in the anus and rectum are called hemorrhoids. They may occur externally or internally. They must be ligated and ligatured after the sphincter of the anus is dilated.
(2:329)

51. **(B)** The padded footboard is used, depending on the degree of tilt, to keep the patient from sliding down on the table and to maintain foot support.
(2:217)

52. **(C)** Cholecystostomy is performed to permit drainage of the gallbladder or removal of stones. This procedure is generally chosen for acute, poor surgical risk patients.
(32:188)

53. **(A)** Paralytic ileus is loss of tone in the small intestines, causing lack of peristalsis which results in pain and swelling of the abdomen.
(7:789)

54. **(D)** Blunt dissection, using a Kitner or peanut, is employed when removing the gallbladder from the infundibulum to the fundal region.
(11:235)

55. **(C)** Following closure of the incision and dressing application, the legs are fully wrapped with cotton elastic bandages for compression. Early ambulation prevents thrombosis and stimulates circulation.
(2:331)

56. **(B)** The Franklin-Silverman biopsy needle consists of a 14-gauge, thin-wall outer cannula with a beveled obturator. It has an inner split needle that fits into the outer cannula and protrudes beyond the end of it. The distal tips of this split are grooved; they catch tissue in the split as it is withdrawn.
(2:297)

57. **(B)** A guillotine amputation is regarded as an emergency procedure. A second operation is required to close the wound. Patients who are severely ill or toxic or have experienced severe trauma are candidates for this operation.
(2:232)

58. **(B)** The light intensity is high, yet cool. A minimum rise in temperature of the tissues exposed to this light may occur.
(2:298)

59. **(C)** The fundus of the gallbladder is grasped with an Allis or Babcock clamp and the proposed opening is encircled with a purse-string suture; a trocar is then placed in and the contents of the gallbladder are aspirated.
(32:188)

60. **(A)** During a cholecystectomy reperitonealization of the liver bed is accomplished using interrupted or continuous fine chromic suture.
(32:187)

61. **(B)** Dysphagia, or difficult swallowing, is the most common symptom of esophageal disease. It usually develops late in the course of the disease.
(32:210)

62. **(C)** Large, heavy, tapered needles are essential for closure of liver tissue. They have a blunt point which is less apt to puncture a vessel.
(32:197)

63. **(C)** A gastrointestinal setup is not to be added unless bypass into the jejunum is considered.   *(32:182, 183)*

64. **(B)** The groin area contains the superficial group of muscles, the obliques, and Scarpa's fascia. An inguinal herniorrhapy requires incision of Scarpa's fascia.
(32:152)

65. **(C)** Portocaval shunt is indicated in all of the pathologies listed except portal hypotension. It may be done in the presence of moderate degrees of hypersplenism, particularly in patients in whom congestive splenomegaly is of relatively short duration.   *(30:652)*

66. **(C)** If more exposure is needed on a subcostal incision the rectus abdominus muscle is either retracted back or transected.   *(32:149)*

67. **(B)** On the appropriate side of the paramedian rectus incision can be used for intra-abdominal surgery. It is made parallel and about 4 cm lateral to the midline.
(32:148)

68. **(D)** Incarcerated hernias, those whose abdominal contents can no longer be returned successfully to the free abdomen, are in great danger of becoming strangulated. The tissue then becomes ischemic and eventually the contents of the sac will necrose (die).
(32:152)

B. GYNECOLOGIC PROCEDURES

69. **(C)** The internal branches of the common iliac artery are the major blood supply of the pelvis, assisted by the median sacral, rectal, and ovarian arteries and branches of the aorta.   *(32:310)*

70. **(B)** The outer layer of the ovary is known as the cortex. The cortex contains graafian follicles in different stages of maturity. After ovulation, reorganization of the graafian follicles develops the corpus luteum, which is responsible for the production of progesterone, essential for implant of the fertilized ovum.
(32:308)

71. **(B)** The outer surfaces of the fallopian tubes are covered by peritoneum as is the uterus.   *(32:308)*

72. **(C)** The external female organs are known collectively as the vulva. The vulva occupies the central portion of the perineal region.   *(32:309)*

73. **(C)** An applicator is used to paint the cervix with Schiller's solution (iodide). A mahogany brown color covering the entire surface indicates a negative reaction between the iodine and the normal cells of the cervix. If there are any abnormal or immature cells present, the tissue at that spot will not take stain. This test is then positive for malignancy and biopsies must be done.   *(7:963)*

74. **(C)** Myomectomy is usually done on young women with symptoms that indicate the presence of benign tumors who wish to preserve fertility.   *(32:326)*

75. **(B)** Pelvic exenteration is the treatment of choice for recurrent or persistent carcinoma of the cervix. It is considered only after a thorough investigation of the patient and the disease.   *(32:339)*

76. **(C)** In a hysterosalpingogram the tip of a catheter is inserted into the cervical canal and a water-soluble radiopaque dye is instilled. The contrast medium ascends into the corpus uteri and tubes, and yields information about the structure and function of the reproductive organs.   *(2:342)*

77. **(D)** All of the other choices are viable methods to create sterility. Culdoscopy cannot be used for this purpose.   *(32:343)*

78. **(A)** A radical vulvectomy involves abdominal, perineal, and groin dissection; it requires a double setup.
(32:317)

79. **(C)** A Wullstein retractor is a small self-retaining retractor used in ENT surgery. All of the others may be used in abdominal pelvic surgery.   *(32:315)*

80. **(C)** The external lateral ligament is a ligament of the knee joint. The broad, round, uterosacral, and cardinal are suspensory ligaments of the uterus.   *(32:319)*

81. **(A)** The abdominal cavity and the fallopian tube are sites of extrauterine pregnancies (ectopic). A salpingostomy done in the early stages of pregnancy may preserve the tube.   *(7:977)*

82. **(B)** Adenomyosis has certain features similar to endometriosis and is sometimes referred to as internal endometriosis. It is characterized by benign invasion of the myometrium by the endometrium.   *(38:725)*

83. **(C)** A Foley catheter is inserted into a presurgical hysterectomy patient to proved constant bladder drainage and prevent trauma to the bladder.   *(32:335)*

84. **(A)** Cystoceles (bulging bladder) and rectoceles (bulging rectum) occur due to weakened vaginal mucosa. Usually the cause is traumatic childbirth and the cure is an anterior and posterior vaginal repair.
(17:266)

85. **(B)** Trachelorrhaphy is done to treat deep lacerations of the cervix and reconstruct the cervical canal.
(32:325)

86. **(C)** Episiotomy is an intentionally made perineal incision executed during a normal birth to facilitate delivery and prevent perineal laceration. *(14:82)*

87. **(A)** Carcinoma-in-situ (stage 0) is limited to the epithelial layer with no evidence of invasion. Surgical treatment is conization of the cervix when fertility is to be preserved; hysterectomy is performed when fertility is not a consideration. *(7:993)*

88. **(C)** Cervical carcinoma has an incidence ratio of 3 to 1 over other reproductive malignancies. It is almost always curable in its preinvasive stage, therefore, early diagnosis is important. *(7:992)*

89. **(C)** Retroversion or retroflexion is the backward displacement of the uterus. It gives rise to backache, pelvic pressure, and fatigue. The only surgical treatment is to reposition the uterus and shorten the support ligaments. *(7:989)*

90. **(B)** Aspiration of fluid or blood from the cul-de-sac of Douglas (culdocentesis) confirms intraperitoneal bleeding due to ectopic pregnancy. *(7:977)*

91. **(B)** Salpingostomy, or tuboplasty, is removal of the obstructed portion of a fallopian tube and opening of the remaining portion of the tube for possibility of fertilization. *(32:343)*

92. **(C)** Bartholin's glands are homologous to the bulbourethral glands (Cowper's) in the male. They are located on either side of the vagina in the labia majora. *(32:310)*

93. **(B)** Functional cysts comprise the majority of ovarian enlargements. Follicle cysts are the most common. *(32:342)*

94. **(D)** An enterocele almost always contains a loop of small intestine which has slipped into the vaginal vault at the cul-de-sac. *(32:320)*

95. **(C)** A Marshall-Marchetti procedure is an abdominal approach to repairing the fascial and the pubococcygeal muscle surrounding the urethra and the bladder neck. *(32:324)*

96. **(A)** A vesicovaginal fistula, one that occurs between the bladder and the vagina, is the most common type. Severity of the fistula may be from small seepage to full voiding into the vagina. *(2:344)*

97. **(C)** Direct visualization of pelvic organs and adjacent structures through a culdoscope, which is introduced into the peritoneal cavity via the pouch of Douglas, is called culdoscopy. *(2:340)*

98. **(B)** Papanicolaou is a cytologic study of smears of the cervical and endocervical tissue. Characteristic cellular changes can be identified. *(2:340)*

99. **(B)** Menstruation is the periodic discharge of blood, mucus, disintegrated ovum, and uterine mucosa formed during the cycle. *(2:338)*

100. **(D)** Kraske position is modification of prone position and is used for rectal procedures. It is also termed the jackknife position. *(32:97–98)*

101. **(C)** Some stirrups may require padding between the calves of the leg and the post. Pressure against soft tissue may predispose to venous thrombus. *(32:96)*

102. **(C)** Metrorrhagia is abnormal bleeding at irregular intervals, either between menses or postmenopausal. *(6:667)*

103. **(A)** The position used to effect a laparoscopy is a lithotomy position. The use of stirrups which do not compromise access to the abdominal area is important. *(32:333)*

104. **(D)** A 1 cm incision is placed below or to the left of the umbilicus. It is easily closed with one or two sutures after the trocar sheath has been removed. *(32:333)*

C. EYE, EAR, NOSE, THROAT, AND PLASTIC SURGERY

105. **(A)** Mydriatics dilate the pupil while allowing the patient to focus. A cycloplegic drug also can dilate the pupil but it disturbs focusing ability. *(33:125)*

106. **(C)** The cryoprobe is attached to the upper anterior surface of the cataract, taking care that it does not adhere to the iris or the cornea. The cryoprobe adheres to the cataract by freezing to its surface. *(33:125)*

107. **(D)** Since it causes no symptoms, early detection of glaucoma is possible only by routine measurement of the eye pressure with a tonometer. Use of eyedrops can prevent this kind of blindness, if started early. *(33:118)*

108. **(C)** A delicate transparent framework called the vitreous humor occupies the inside of the back part of the eye. In the older eye the vitreous framework shrinks; if attached to the retina it causes a tear and the retina then detaches. *(33:129)*

109. **(B)** The instrument used to measure intraocular pressure is a tonometer. A number of types are available. When placed on the cornea, a tonometer causes corneal indentation, the amount of which depends on the intraocular pressure. *(33:59)*

110. **(C)** Ectropion is the sagging and eversion of the lower lid. It is common in older patients and is corrected by a plastic procedure which shortens the lower lid in a horizontal direction.   *(32:667)*

111. **(C)** Enucleation is removal of the entire eyeball. Evisceration is removal of the contents of the eye, leaving the sclera intact.   *(32:676)*

112. **(B)** Creation of a tract lined with iris tissue, which serves as a wick to accomplish filtration (thus reducing the abnormal pressure of glaucoma), is called iridencleisis.   *(32:688)*

113. **(B)** Resection of part of the ocular muscle rotates the eye toward the operated muscle and thereby strengthens it.   *(32:672)*

114. **(C)** In its normal state, the vitreous gel of the eye is transparent. In certain disease states it becomes opaque and must be removed.   *(32:682)*

115. **(C)** When performing a stapedectomy, very fine hooks with 45-, 90-, and 180-degree angles are essential dissecting tools.   *(32:599)*

116. **(A)** Incision of the tympanic membrane, known as myringotomy, is done to treat otitis media. By releasing the fluid behind the membrane, hearing is restored and infection controlled. Frequently, tubes are inserted through the tympanic membrane.   *(32:603)*

117. **(C)** An endaural fenestration procedure is done to restore hearing in persons with otosclerosis of the tympanic membrane and ossicles. The objective is to create a new permanent window through which sound waves can enter the inner ear when the oval window is fixed.   *(32:609)*

118. **(C)** Stapes mobilization (stapediolysis) is re-establishment of a functioning linkage between the incus and the inner ear. Stapediolysis means removal (or lysis) of bony or fibrous adhesions around the stapes.   *(32:612)*

119. **(D)** When a mass of adenoid obstructs the pharyngeal orifice of the eustachian tube, a partial vacuum forms, causing serum to fill the tympanic cavity. Treatment is adenoidectomy.   *(33:414)*

120. **(D)** In dealing with hearing loss, the loudness is measured in decibels (db). It is a logarithmic method of dealing with large numbers.   *(32:591)*

121. **(A)** Seldom seen today, mastoiditis was a common complication of the preantibiotic era. It still occurs, but less frequently and less severely because most patients receive antibiotics and stop the disease process early.   *(33:401)*

122. **(D)** Otoplasty is the correct term for "earpinning." It is a simple surgical procedure frequently done on small children before adult psychologic trauma can occur.   *(2:214)*

123. **(C)** The cochlea, located in the inner ear with the labyrinth, is involved in the sense of hearing. The labyrinth (composed of the utricle, saccule, and semicircular canals) is responsible for equilibrium.   *(32:590)*

124. **(C)** Aural, as used in endaural: through the ear canal, or postaural: outside the ear canal.   *(33:374)*

125. **(C)** Sound waves collect in the auricle, the outer ear, and are transmitted into the external canal to hit the eardrum (tympanic membrane).   *(32:590)*

126. **(A)** Adenoid tissue located at the roof of the nasopharynx is often the cause of blockage in the eustachian tube, causing otitis media. This procedure is a pediatric procedure since adenoid tissue atrophies after adolescence.   *(2:417)*

127. **(B)** The Ballinger swivel knife is used with a septal elevator to elevate the mucous membrane away from the cartilage during a submucous resection.   *(32:621)*

128. **(B)** Removal of either the cartilaginous or osseous portions of the septum that lie between the flaps of the mucous membrane and perichondrium is called a submucous resection of the septum.   *(32:621)*

129. **(C)** Epistaxis (nosebleed) generally comes from the anterior portion of the nasal septum, where there is a plexus of tiny arteries and veins called Kiesselback's plexus.   *(33:245)*

130. **(B)** Once the nasal bone or upper lateral cartilage is fractured, the deformity (hump) on the bone and possibly the septal cartilage are removed by the Jansen-Middleton forceps, osteotomes, a mallet, and scissors.   *(32:621–622)*

131. **(C)** Mediastinoscopy requires a short transverse incision directly above the suprasternal notch. The scope is then inserted for viewing.   *(32:370)*

132. **(C)** The Potts tissue forceps is a fine forceps associated with vascular and fine intestinal surgery. Nasal surgery requires, intranasally, an angled forceps such as the bayonet forceps, a Freer elevator, and a fine Frazier suction tube.   *(32:622–623)*

133. **(C)** Frequently a topical anesthetic is used prior to nasal surgery. The drug of choice is cocaine, 10% or 4%, and would be administered by means of soaked applicators introduced into the nasal cavity and absorbed by the mucous membrane.   *(2:179; 32:616)*

134. **(C)** The ethmoid sinus lies bilaterally between the nose and the orbits. The maxillary sinuses are below them and the frontal sinuses are above them.

    (32:613–614)

135. **(C)** Tracheostomy is the opening of the trachea and establishment of a new airway through a midline incision in the neck, below the cricoid cartilage. A cannula is put in place to maintain the airway. This is an emergency procedure.   *(32:644)*

136. **(B)** Most tracheostomy tubes consist of three parts: the outer cannula, the inner cannula, and the obturator. The inner cannula is periodically removed for cleansing but must be replaced immediately to prevent the outer cannula from crusting, which would cause an obstruction.   *(2:427)*

137. **(A)** This surgery is indicated in carcinoma of the epiglottis and false cords, which are located distally to the true cords. It preserves phonotory, respiratory, and sphincteric functions of the larynx.   *(32:648)*

138. **(C)** Most neoplasms of the salivary glands are benign mixed tumors; most of these affect the parotid gland.

    (33:223)

139. **(D)** Dacrocystorhinostomy creates a new larger opening between the lacrimal sac and the nasal sinus in persons with chronic dacrocystitis where tear ducts are blocked.   *(17:445)*

140. **(A)** Otosclerosis is a condition characterized by deafness, caused by the formation of spongy bone, especially around the oval window with resulting ankylosis of the stapes.   *(36:1192)*

141. **(B)** The adult patient is placed in semi-Fowler's or Fowler's position, with the surgeon sitting directly in front. Local anesthesia is frequently used.   *(2:422)*

142. **(D)** A Cottle cartilage holder would be found on a setup for nasal surgery. All of the others are tonsillectomy instruments.   *(32:638)*

143. **(B)** To maintain hemostasis postoperatively in radical neck surgery, a Hemovac is generally employed. Continuous pressure from the gauze pressure dressings reduces the accumulation of serosanguineous fluid, which is removed by the Hemovac.   *(32:649, 654)*

144. **(A)** Glossectomy is removal of the tongue, and frequently the floor of the mouth.   *(2:421)*

145. **(A)** A split thickness graft, or partial thickness graft, contains epidermis and only a portion of the dermis.   *(2:447)*

146. **(A)** Dupuytren's contracture is a progressive disease involving the palmar fascia and the digital extensions of the palmar fascia. The surgery required is a palmar fasciectomy.   *(32:583)*

147. **(C)** The patient's age, the size of extremity, and the patient's systolic pressure are all factors to be considered when applying a tourniquet. The depth of the incision is of no consequence.   *(32:576)*

148. **(B)** A limb is exsanguinated by progressively wrapping from the distal phalanges to the tourniquet cuff with an Esmarch rubber bandage. The limb is then elevated until exsanguination is accomplished. The tourniquet is then inflated and the bandage removed.

    (32:576)

149. **(B)** Microtia refers to congenital total or subtotal absence of the external ear.   *(32:554)*

150. **(C)** The Stryker instrument is pneumatic-powered; it uses as its power source a nonflammable, inert gas. It operates saws, dermatatoo machines, and the dermabrader. The Reese and the Padgett-Hood are drum-type dermatomes. The Brown is a motor-driven dermatome.   *(32:533, 534)*

151. **(D)** Nonadherence to tissue is a great advantage when using silicone implants.   *(32:531)*

152. **(B)** The pedicle flap is left attached to the donor site to maintain viability of the flap.   *(32:543)*

153. **(B)** Most fractures of the body of the mandible occur in patients with teeth, and can be managed by closed reduction and intramaxillary fixation with arch bars and rubber bands.   *(29:300)*

154. **(C)** Prognathism, a forward jutting of the jaw, and micrognathia, an abnormally small jaw, are corrected surgically by a mentoplasty.   *(2:450)*

155. **(A)** The patient is placed in a semi-Fowler's position or on one side, horizontally to prevent aspiration of blood or venous engorgement. Head is turned to the side.   *(32:638)*

156. **(C)** During the harvesting of skin for a split thickness graft, the donor site is pulled taut with a tongue depressor allowing the dermatome to slide easily.

    (17:388)

D. GENITOURINARY PROCEDURES

157. **(B)** As the male ages, the prostate gland may enlarge and gradually obstruct the urethra. This condition is known as benign prostatic hypertrophy (BPH).
(7:1032)

158. **(B)** Large strictures can be readily dilated by the use of Van Buren sounds. These metal sounds are curved to approximate the general curvature of the male urethra. *(18:36)*

159. **(A)** A stone may lodge in a renal calyx and continue to enlarge, eventually filling the entire calyx or renal pelvis. It is known as a staghorn stone. *(32:385)*

160. **(D)** The cortex of the adrenal glands secretes hormones on which various tumors are dependent. Bilateral adrenalectomy restricts further growth of the tumor. *(32:299)*

161. **(D)** A nephrostomy is accomplished by temporarily draining the kidney with a Malecot or Pezzar catheter. *(32:289)*

162. **(C)** All of the instruments mentioned are required to remove a rib except a Heaney clamp, which is a hemostatic clamp used in gynecologic surgery. *(32:286)*

163. **(B)** Epispadias is the condition in which the urethral meatus is situated abnormally on the upper side of the penis. This is opposed to hypospadias, where the opening is abnormally located on the underside of the penis. *(32:260)*

164. **(B)** Removal of the testes (orchiectomy) renders the patient both sterile and hormone deficient. Bilateral orchiectomy usually denotes carcinoma. Unilateral orchiectomy may be indicated for cancer, infection, or trauma. *(32:271)*

165. **(C)** All of the incisions are optional for kidney removal except Kocher's incision, which is applicable to biliary surgery. *(32:285)*

166. **(C)** Here the pelvis of the kidney is incised with a small blade. A catheter is placed through the incision into the renal penis to create a urinary diversion. *(32:289)*

167. **(C)** The resectoscope has five components: the sheath, the obturator, the telescope, the working element, and the cutting electrode. The lithotrite is an instrument used through a cystoscope to crush or pulverize calculi. *(2:363)*

168. **(B)** Conductive lubricants must never be used on the sheath of a resectoscope. They may provide a pathway for an electrical current. *(2:363)*

169. **(B)** All are examples of cystoscopes except the Stern-McCarthy, which is a resectoscope (an instrument used to excise tissue from the bladder, urethra, and prostate). *(2:363)*

170. **(C)** Recannulization of the vas deferens for restoration of fertility requires nonobstructed anastomosis, called a vasovasostomy. *(2:359)*

171. **(B)** An anastomosis, usually between the radial artery and the cephalic vein in the forearm, creates an arteriolized peripheral vein that permits dialysis connections to be made for venipuncture. This is called an arteriovenous fistula. *(2:353)*

172. **(C)** The Quinton-Scribner shunt, the oldest and simplest device, consists of two Teflon tips attached to a silastic tubing. One is placed in the artery, the other in the vein. Connecting tubing is exteriorized. This provides ready access to a patient's circulation for hemodialysis. *(2:353)*

173. **(C)** To "harvest a kidney" is to remove a kidney from a cadaver for transplant. Meticulous dissection is necessary to free the kidney, its blood vessels, and the ureter with minimal trauma. *(2:352)*

174. **(D)** Hemodialysis is the process of removing waste products from the blood of a patient in renal failure by diffusion through a semipermeable membrane of a dialyzer (artificial kidney machine). *(2:353)*

175. **(B)** Following a TUR, the urologist may insert a 30-cc, 3-way Foley catheter. The third lumen provides a means of continuous irrigation of the bladder for a period after surgery to prevent the formation of clots. *(2:359)*

176. **(D)** The suprapubic approach is limited almost exclusively to removal of a large, benign hypertrophied gland over 50 grams in weight. *(2:359)*

177. **(C)** In accomplishing a retropubic prostatectomy, the gland is exposed through a transverse or vertical abdominal incision above the symphysis pubis. The gland is removed through an incision in the prostate capsule. This procedure is also called a transcapsular prostatectomy. *(2:360)*

178. **(B)** Nephrosclerosis is hardening or sclerosis of the arteries of the kidney and is usually seen secondary to renal hypertension. *(7:935)*

179. **(B)** Pyelonephrosis is a disease of the pelvis of the kidney. It is usually due to bacteria that have ascended from the bladder after entrance through the urethra. *(36:142)*

180. **(B)** If a stone is in the kidney, the abdominal operation performed is a nephrolithotomy, or a simple incision into the kidney and stone removal.   *(7:942)*

181. **(D)** Orchiopexy is regarded as the transfer or fixation of an imperfectly descended testicle into the scrotum and suturing it in place.   *(36:1172)*

182. **(B)** After a suprapubic incision is made abdominally, an opening is made into the bladder and the prostate is removed from above.   *(32:276)*

183. **(C)** Postoperative epididymitis is a complication of prostatectomy. The infection passes upward through the urethra, and thence along the vas deferens to the epididymis.   *(7:1030)*

184. **(D)** Seminal fluid is manufactured in the seminal vesicles and the prostate gland.   *(7:1030)*

185. **(A)** Early diagnosis of scrotal pain can reverse torsion of the spermatic cord and reduce the possibility of loss of the testicle.   *(26:447)*

186. **(D)** Hydroureter refers to the distention of the ureter with fluid due to an obstruction distal to the distention.   *(36:791)*

187. **(C)** Glycine, which is isosmotic and nonelectrolytic, is generally used during transurethral surgery. Water may be used for cystoscopy but is contraindicated for TUR because it is hypotonic.   *(18:17)*

188. **(B)** Meatal stenosis in the male is usually the result of inflammation (balanitis, urethritis). The surgical correction is a meatotomy.   *(26:404)*

189. **(C)** The principle of lithotripsy consists of an electronic circuitry that generates a series of low-amp, high-voltage, direct-current impulses sparking across the tip of a coaxial electrode. When the electrode is located in a liquid medium, the energy produces a shock wave that fragments a calculus.   *(18:300)*

190. **(A)** Indications for palliative upper urinary tract diversion remain controversial. The pigtail stent and the Gibbons catheter provide palliative diversion in patients with malignant obstruction.   *(18:287)*

191. **(A)** Surgical removal of the foreskin of the penis is frequently removed immediately after birth. At times the condition known as phimosis (stricture of the foreskin) causes a circumcision to be done on an adult male who was not circumcised at birth.   *(17:285)*

E. THORACIC, CARDIOVASCULAR, AND PERIPHERAL VASCULAR PROCEDURES

192. **(B)** The thoraseal unit is one of the disposable Pleuravacs or chest drainage units. It is a three-chamber unit which closely resembles the three-bottle system. Raising the unit above the level of the bed will increase intrathoracic pressure and collapse the lung. The air inlet in the third chamber must remain unobstructed.   *(31:40)*

193. **(C)** Cardiac catheterization is utilized to diagnose coronary artery disease. It involves a sterile setup and fluoroscopy to diagnose ischemic heart disease. The brachial or femoral artery is used to effect this procedure.   *(2:391)*

194. **(D)** The sternum is reattached with heavy-gauge stainless steel sutures. The resultant complication can be brachial plexus injury and costochondrial separation from too vigorous retraction in surgery.   *(2:384)*

195. **(C)** Air and blood in the pleural cavity may be detected and aspirated with a needle and syringe; this is called thoracentesis. If bleeding continues, the chest must be opened.   *(2:388)*

196. **(C)** The scalene nodes, used diagnostically for detecting malignancy of the lung, are approached via a supraclavicular incision.   *(32:67)*

197. **(B)** A reduction of negative pressure on one side causes the negative pressure on the normal side to pull on the mediastinum in an effort to equalize the pressure. This is referred to as mediastinal shift; it tends to compress the lung, causing dyspnea.   *(32:353)*

198. **(C)** Removal of the fibrinous deposit or restrictive membrane on the visceral and parietal pleura that interferes with pulmonary function is called decortication of the lung.   *(32:374)*

199. **(A)** After the muscle attachments of the rib are removed, the rib is excised with a bone shear and the rough edges are trimmed with a Stille-Luer rongeur. Bone wax may be used for hemostasis.   *(32:372)*

200. **(B)** If a stapling instrument is to be used to resect a wedge of lung, the TA 55 will be used. The instrument is applied to one side of the wedge, shot, reloaded, and applied to the other side. A scalpel is used to dissect the wedge from between the adjoining rows of staples.   *(32:371)*

201. **(C)** The Lovelace lung-grasping forceps is used to grasp and immobilize the lung prior to surgical inspection and surgery.   *(32:371)*

202. **(B)** The patent ductus arteriosis is an important fetal vascular communication, whereby blood is shunted from the pulmonary artery to the aorta (because the lungs are nonfunctioning) and the blood is oxygenated by the placenta. Closure of the patent ductus arteriosis is accomplished surgically if the opening has not closed by itself after birth. *(32:418)*

203. **(C)** The Satinsky vena cava clamp, the Rumel tourniquet, and the Potts cardiovascular scissors would all be found on the setup. The Allen clamp is an intestinal noncrushing clamp. *(32:389)*

204. **(D)** Cardiac patches, heart valves, and tubular grafts are made of Teflon, Dacron, and silicone rubber. Additionally, porcine heterografts (aortic valves of a pig) are used. *(32:391)*

205. **(C)** Choices A, B, and D are the three components of a cardiopulmonary bypass system. To restart the heart after surgery the need for a ventricular fibrillator would be additional. *(32:385–386)*

206. **(C)** Perfusion is the technique of oxygenating and perfusing the blood by means of a mechanical pump-oxygenator. *(2:392)*

207. **(D)** Endarterectomy is the removal of arteriosclerotic plaque from an obstructed artery. It occurs frequently at the bifurcation of the vessel. *(17:401)*

208. **(C)** The most frequent underlying condition requiring a permanent pacemaker is heart block, in which there is a disturbance of the neuroconductive system. *(32:422)*

209. **(B)** The electrode is inserted through a small incision in the external jugular or cephalic vein, where its course goes into the superior vena cava. It is then positioned at the apex of the right ventricle. *(12:203)*

210. **(C)** A venotomy is done through a small incision with a #11 blade and Potts scissors. The electrode is then threaded into the left ventricle by visualization through an image intensifier fluoroscope, and a pocket is made to hold the pacemaker with a tunneling instrument. The pacemaker is placed into the pocket in the chest and attached to the electrode. *(32:422)*

211. **(C)** A, B, and D are optional power sources for pulse generators (pacemakers). *(32:422)*

212. **(B)** Tetralogy of Fallot is the most common congenital cardiac anomaly of the cyanotic group. Physiologically, in tetralogy of Fallot, blood flow into the lungs decreases as a result of pulmonary obstruction, and a right-left shunt of venous blood from the right ventricle to the left ventricle and aorta occurs. This delivers unoxygenated blood through the arterial system; the obstruction must be cleared surgically. *(32:410)*

213. **(D)** For implantation of epicardial electrodes, an extrapleural parasternal approach is one of the several approaches used. The pericardium is entered by subperichondrial resection of the fifth costal cartilage. Either a sew-in or screw-type electrode is implanted in the epicardium of the right or left ventricle. The electrode is then attached to a generator and placed into a subcutaneous pocket in the abdomen or chest wall. *(2:395)*

214. **(C)** Anastomosis of the hepatic artery and the inferior vena cava would devascularize the liver and cause liver necrosis. *(10:236)*

215. **(D)** The dilation of the saphenous vein produces a venous stasis with secondary edema. Repeated attacks of inflammation of these veins would eventually be followed by ulceration and finally gangrene. *(7:645)*

216. **(C)** During an arterial embolectomy a Fogarty catheter is carefully inserted into an artery and placed beyond the point of the clot attachment. The balloon is inflated, and the catheter is withdrawn along with the attached clot. *(32:434)*

217. **(A)** A filter device may be inserted (in its collapsed form) through a cutdown in a large vein, usually the right internal jugular. The Mobbin-Uddin filter is shaped like an umbrella. It is designed to allow blood to pass through the cava while filtering clots. *(11:407)*

218. **(D)** Bulldog clamps are small, spring-like clamps which are noncrushing in nature and are used to occlude peripheral vessels during surgery. *(32:438)*

219. **(D)** An indication for inferior vena cava clipping is the recurrence of pulmonary emboli (after heparinization is deemed inadequate). A Miles Teflon clip is placed around the IVC. After placement of the clip, blood flow is maintained, but massive emboli are prevented from passing into the lungs. *(10:234)*

220. **(C)** A graft placed proximal to and inclusive of the common iliac vessels will necessitate the use of a bifurcation into the common iliac branches. *(32:430)*

221. **(A)** The development of alternate routes of circulation is known as collateral circulation. *(32:426)*

222. **(D)** Surgical removal of sympathetic ganglia (sympathectomy) is indicated for persons with arteriosclerotic peripheral vascular disease. *(10:208)*

223. **(D)** To prevent undue trauma, umbilical tapes or vessel loops are used for retraction and vascular control. *(2:395)*

F. ORTHOPEDICS, PLASTER

224. **(D)** Bone wax is rubbed onto the bleeding stomas of the surface of bone to stop bleeding. *(32:104)*

225. **(A)** Webbing between the fingers is the most common congenital deformity of the hand. Syndactyly (syndactylism) may occur in the foot also. *(2:470)*

226. **(A)** A Lane bone-holding forceps is used to hold shafts of long bones. *(6:116)*

227. **(A)** A Minerva jacket is applied from the hips to the head. If the head is to be completely immobilized, it is included in the jacket. *(2:378)*

228. **(C)** Esmarch bandage is rubber-rolled bandage used to facilitate drainage of vessels for application of a tourniquet. *(2:377)*

229. **(B)** A fracture of the clavicle is usually treated non-surgically by immobilization in a figure-eight splint. *(32:513)*

230. **(B)** A Keller arthroplasty is a variation of a bunionectomy in which the proximal third of the phalynx is excised and replaced by a silicone implant. *(2:375)*

231. **(A)** Baker's cysts, generally found in the popliteal space in children, usually occur without predisposing factors. When found in adults they may be indicative of an intra-articular disease. *(32:518)*

232. **(A)** Ganglia are benign outpouchings of synovium from the intercarpal joints that become filled with synovial fluid. They often resolve spontaneously but occasionally must be excised. *(32:488)*

233. **(B)** In carpal tunnel syndrome the median nerve becomes compressed at the volar surface of the wrist because of thickened synovium, fractures, or aberrant muscles. *(32:487)*

234. **(B)** In young adults chronic dislocation of the patella can be due to a shallow condylar groove and a patella proximal to the normal anatomic position. If this condition persists chondromalacia may occur. *(32:511)*

235. **(B)** A torn meniscus is the most common injury involving the knee joint. An injured meniscus, either medial or lateral, must be removed if torn. The procedure is called a meniscectomy. *(32:517)*

236. **(C)** A derotational osteotomy is performed when there is improper seating of the head of the acetabulum. The femur is placed in internal rotation and is divided. The distal fragment is rotated externally in order to place the knee and foot straight ahead. The patient is then immobilized in a spica cast. *(32:502)*

237. **(D)** A Colle's fracture is the most common and classic fracture. It is caused by breaking a fall with the outstretched hand. *(24:190)*

238. **(C)** A spiral fracture resembles an oblique fracture, differing only in length. *(32:464)*

239. **(D)** If anatomic reduction by manipulation is impossible and nonunion of the femoral neck fracture is apparent, the choice of hardware may be either a Thompson, an Austin-Moore, or a Machett-Brown femoral head prosthetic replacement. *(32:496)*

240. **(B)** Hip reconstruction or total hip replacement is most commonly indicated in patients with hip pain due to rheumatoid arthritis or osteoarthritis. *(32:500)*

241. **(D)** A basic bone set includes a mallet, periosteal elevators, gouges, curettes, bone cutters, osteotomes, rongeurs, and chisels. Drivers and extractors are required only to implant hardward and are considered additional instrumentation. *(32:462)*

242. **(C)** Hammer-toe deformity causes painful calluses on the dorsal joints of the four lateral toes, as the coiled-up digits rest against the shoes. *(32:524)*

243. **(B)** Reconstruction of a joint, arthroplasty, may be necessary to restore or improve range of motion and stability or to relieve pain. *(2:374)*

244. **(A)** The Küntscher, Schneider, and Hansen-Street are all capable of reducing a fracture of the adult femur. The Smith-Petersen nail is used to reduce a fracture of the femoral neck. *(32:505)*

245. **(D)** A Mira reamer is used to ream the acetabulum for replacement of the acetabular cup with a prosthesis. The osteotomes, rongeur, and Gigli saw all aid in removing the femoral head. *(6:205–206)*

246. **(B)** The virulence of osteomyelitis frequently determines the severity of the disease. The most common causative organism is *Staphylococcus;* the next most common is *Streptococcus.* *(24:317)*

247. **(D)** Arthrodesis is most commonly employed to relieve pain by eliminating motion, to provide stability where normal ligament stability has been destroyed, or to correct deformity by realignment at the level of fusion. *(24:377)*

248. **(B)** Scoliosis is either functional and postural (attributable to poor posture and weak musculature or ligaments) or structural, in which there are changes in the shape of the vertebrae. *(24:267)*

249. **(D)** The Minerva jacket, Sayre sling, and Milwaukee brace are capable of correcting slight scoliosis. The Risser jacket and halo traction are used to correct gross deformities, either with or without spinal fusion. *(2:465)*

250. **(B)** Black light, an ultraviolet light in the 3000 to 4000 angstrom range, is used to cure this open-weave fiberglass cast. *(2:379)*

251. **(B)** Talipes varus, the condition known as clubfoot, refers to the inversion of the forefoot. *(2:465)*

252. **(C)** During its acute stage, tuberculous arthritis produces cold abscesses, so named to distinguish them from the acute inflammatory abscesses that are associated with acute infectious disease and which are hot or warm to palpation. *(7:1322)*

253. **(C)** Sequestrum is the dead bone that lines the walls of an abscess cavity resulting from osteomyelitis. *(7:1294)*

254. **(B)** Collagen and ground substance are produced for fracture repair by bone-forming cells called osteoblasts. *(7:1294)*

255. **(A)** Osteoporosis is increased porosity of bone and is responsible for many fractures in the elderly. There is a reduction in the amount of bone mass without a change in chemical composition. *(7:1348)*

256. **(C)** There are five stages of bone healing: hematoma (serves as a fibrin network), cellular proliferation (fibroplastic and endothelial cells colonize fibrin to form clots), callus formation (osteoblasts produce osteoid matrix), callus ossification (this is the union stage), consolidation (the bone is remodeled into mature bone). *(7:1294)*

257. **(B)** Osteoarthritis, the most common of all joint diseases, is degeneration of the articular cartilage in the joints. *(7:1333)*

258. **(A)** A modified wedge osteotomy is the removal of a portion of the vertebrae to allow straightening of the diseased spine. *(7:1336)*

259. **(B)** Multiple myeloma is a malignant disease of plasma cells that infiltrates bone and soft tissue. It occurs characteristically in middle-aged males. *(7:1230)*

260. **(C)** Osteomalacia is a disturbance of calcium and phosphorus metabolism caused by vitamin D deficiency in adults. Severe bony deformities may require surgical intervention. *(7:1347)*

261. **(B)** Harrington rod procedures must include varioussize hex nuts for proper insertion of the rod. These nuts added to the end of the compression rods maintain force against each of the hooks used with the rods. *(6:196)*

262. **(D)** Awl reamers are not necessary for the insertion of Küntscher nails. *(6:156)*

263. **(D)** Cobb elevators are needed only when a spinal fusion is to be done. *(6:192)*

264. **(A)** When preparing plaster rolls or splints they are submerged in warm water (70 to 75°F). When bubbles cease to rise to the surface they are removed, lightly twisted and used. *(2:377)*

265. **(C)** An incomplete fracture, only partly through the bone, is commonly found in children whose bones have not yet calcified. This is a greenstick fracture. *(17:302)*

G. NEUROSURGERY

266. **(D)** Hemostatic scalp clips include Michel, Raney, Adson, and LeRoy clips. *(17:320)*

267. **(B)** Cervical decompression requires postoperative application of Crutchfield tongs for stability of skeletal traction. *(2:440)*

268. **(C)** Cordotomy is the division of the anterolateral column of the spinal pain fibers high in the thoracic or cervical retion. Cordotomy is used most frequently in controlling severe pain of terminal cancer. *(7:1204)*

269. **(B)** The myelogram outlines the spinal subarachnoid space and shows distortions of the spinal cord or dura sac. *(7:1274)*

270. **(D)** Increased intracranial pressure constitutes a true emergency. Body responses include vomiting, changed vital signs, and reduced responsiveness. Increasing pressure produces pupillary changes; their unequal reaction to light would be noted on physical exam. *(7:1185)*

271. **(C)** Hemorrhage in the substance of the brain is most common in patients with high arterial blood pressure and cerebral atherosclerosis. *(7:1184)*

272. **(B)** The term autonomic refers to biologic operations that are independent of the desires and wishes of the individual. This system includes heart muscle, the secretions of all digestive and sweat glands, and the activity of certain endocrine organs as well.
(7:1171)

273. **(C)** A meningioma, arising from the covering of the brain, is an escapsulated, well-defined tumor growing outside the brain and compressing rather than invading the brain.
(32:752)

274. **(B)** Among his many accomplishments Cushing, the father of modern neurosurgery, described the relationship of intracranial pressure to blood pressure in 1900. In 1932 he described pituitary basophilism, commonly known as Cushing's syndrome.
(2:241)

275. **(C)** A subdural hematoma, one which occurs between the dura and the arachnoid, is usually caused by a laceration of the veins that cross the subdural space.
(2:438)

276. **(D)** Neurolysis is the freeing of an adhesed nerve to restore function and relieve pain. Carpal tunnel syndrome is an example in which the median nerve is entrapped in the carpal tunnel of the wrist.
(2:442)

277. **(A)** Cryosurgery utilizes subfreezing temperatures to create a lesion in the treatment of disease, such as Parkinson's disease. This brain lesion destroys diseased cells of the brain and reduces the tremors associated with the disease.
(32:760)

278. **(D)** Suboccipital craniectomy for posterior fossa exploration involves perforation and removal of the posterior occipital bone and exposure of the foramen magnum and arch of the atlas.
(32:756)

279. **(C)** A newborn anomaly which is represented by incomplete closure of the vertebral arches, with or without herniation of the meninges, is called spina bifida.
(2:469)

280. **(D)** Bipolar units are commonly used in neurosurgery. They provide a completely isolated output with negligi-

ble leakage of current between the tips of the forceps, permitting use of coagulation current in proximity to structures where ordinary unipolar coagulation would be hazardous.
(32:729)

281. **(B)** Schwartz temporary vascular clamps can be removed after application.
(32:744)

282. **(C)** A Selverstone carotid artery clamp for gradual occlusion of the carotid artery is necessary for the setup. The other clamps are vascular clips for cranial aneurysms.
(32:772)

283. **(B)** A Cloward procedure is done to relieve pain in the neck, shoulder, or arm caused by cervical spondylosis or herniated disk. It involves removal of the disk with fusion of the vertebral bodies.
(32:770)

284. **(C)** In craniosynostosis the suture line of an infant has closed prematurely. A synthetic material (such as silicone) is used to keep the edges of the cranial sutures from reuniting and preventing brain growth.
(32:757)

285. **(C)** Hemostatic scalp clips include Michele clips, Raney clips, or Adson clips. Raney and Adson are reusable; they are removed at the time of closure of the skin flap and rewashed. The Raney and Michele clips are hand loaded and must be reshaped after use. The Heifitz clip is an aneurysm clip used for cranial aneurysms.
(32:725)

286. **(A)** Preparation for neurosurgery should include preoperative arrangements with the anesthesiologist for the management of a possible air embolus.
(32:723)

287. **(A)** Surgical trauma to the first and second cranial nerves would cause loss of the senses of smell and sight.
(32:749)

288. **(C)** After burr holes have been created with a perforator, the bone may be cut between the holes with a flexible multifilament wire (Gigli saw) or air-powered craniotome.
(2:434)

Practice Test

**CAREFULLY READ THE FOLLOWING INSTRUCTIONS
BEFORE TAKING THE PRACTICE TEST**

1. This exam consists of 250 questions. You will be required to take the entire exam in 3 hours. As on the Certifying Examination, this gives you an average of 40 to 45 seconds per question.
2. Be certain to have an adequate number of pencils and erasers with you.
3. Schedule the test to be taken in a quiet, *uninterrupted* atmosphere. Be certain a clock is in sight to help you pace yourself.
4. Remove the answer grid from pages 181 and 182 and fill out properly.
5. Be certain that the number on the answer sheet corresponds to the question number on the test.
6. When the test is completed, compare the responses with those supplied at the end of the test section.
7. An additional sheet has been provided at the end of the test section that identifies which questions are reflective of a particular subject.
8. Additional study emphasis may be required in a particular area if you have not correctly completed at least 75% of the identified questions on a particular subject.

Questions

1. In an inguinal herniorrhaphy the spermatic cord is

   A. ligated with a hemoclip
   B. retracted with a Penrose drain
   C. incised for ease of access
   D. clamped with a Kelly

2. Polyglycolic acid sutures are

   A. absorbed by an enzyme action
   B. absorbed by the process of hydrolysis
   C. nonabsorbable
   D. encapsulated by body tissue

3. The pounds of pressure necessary in a flash steam sterilizer set at 270°F is

   A. 15
   B. 17
   C. 20
   D. 27

4. Connie H. is having elective surgery. The nurse notes that her white cell count is 14,000 cu mm. This would indicate that

   A. there may be an inflammation or infection present and surgery could be cancelled until it is further investigated
   B. the count is within normal range and surgery can proceed
   C. there may be an inflammation or infection present
   D. there may be an anemic condition present and surgery should be cancelled

5. The suffix *itis* means

   A. condition
   B. pain
   C. inflammation
   D. study of

6. Meckel's diverticulum is found in the

   A. esophagus
   B. sigmoid colon
   C. ileum
   D. duodenum

7. Use of a Frazier suction requires the presence of a/an

   A. adapter
   B. trocar
   C. stylette
   D. obturator

8. Airborne contamination is reduced by recirculation of filtered outside air at a rate of

   A. 12 air exchanges per minute
   B. 12 air exchanges per hour
   C. 20 air exchanges per minute
   D. 25 air exchanges per hour

9. Slander is

   A. an oral derogatory statement about a physician's competence
   B. a discussion of a patient's condition outside of the OR
   C. an unlawful threat of harm
   D. a physical threat of harm

10. Without is symbolized by

    A. w/o
    B. aa
    C. $\bar{c}$
    D. $\bar{s}$

11. If a family is contacted but cannot come in to sign a permission for emergency surgery, the surgeon would

A. work without permission
B. accept permission by phone, telegram, or in writing
C. ask another physician to sign
D. refuse to do the case

12. Unwrapped instruments are sterilized at 270°F (132°C) for a minimum of

A. 3 minutes
B. 5 minutes
C. 7 minutes
D. 10 minutes

13. A retention suture does *not* pass through

A. mesentery tissue
B. rectus muscle
C. fascial tissue
D. subcutaneous tissue

14. A hernia that passes through the inguinal ring into the inguinal canal is termed

A. direct
B. indirect
C. pantaloon
D. sliding

15. Dead space is the space

A. that has no blood supply
B. caused by separation of wound edges that have not been closely approximated
C. where the tissue has been approximated with sutures
D. where the suture line has broken down

16. Unwrapped tubing can be sterilized in a high-speed sterilizer at 270°F for a minimum of

A. 3 minutes
B. 5 minutes
C. 10 minutes
D. 15 minutes

17. Special stockings or elastic bandages may be ordered to the lower extremities prior to surgery to

A. provide comfort to the patient
B. prevent postural hypotension
C. provide vasoconstriction of lower extremities
D. prevent thrombophlebitis or embolus formation

18. Which term denotes low or decreased blood volume?

A. anoxia
B. hypovolemia
C. hypoxia
D. hypocapnia

19. Injection of contrast media into the brachial, carotid, or vertebral artery to study the intracranial vessels is called

A. myelography
B. pneumoencephalography
C. CAT scan
D. angiography

20. Instruments and tubing sterilized together in the flash autoclave require

A. 3 minutes at 270°F
B. 53 minutes at 250°F
C. 10 minutes at 270°F
D. 30 minutes at 250°F

21. Suture material that becomes encapsulated with fibrous tissue during the healing process is

A. nonabsorbable suture
B. absorbable suture
C. synthetic absorbable suture
D. gut suture

22. A right hemicolectomy is performed to remove pathology of the

A. descending colon
B. ascending colon
C. sigmoid colon
D. mesocolon

23. Adduction means

A. movement away from the median plane
B. movement toward the median plane
C. movement superiorly
D. movement inferiorly

24. When transporting a patient, drainage systems should be placed

A. at stretcher level
B. below stretcher level
C. above stretcher level
D. optionally

25. The maximum size of a linen pack must not exceed

A. 8 × 10 × 16 inches
B. 10 × 14 × 18 inches
C. 12 × 12 × 20 inches
D. 14 × 16 × 36 inches

26. Another name for a stay suture is a/an

A. tension suture
B. retention suture
C. interrupted suture
D. buried suture

27. What two anatomic structures are ligated and divided to effect a cholecystectomy?

A. common hepatic duct, common bile duct
B. cystic duct, cystic artery
C. common bile duct, cystic artery
D. cystic duct, hepatic artery

28. Puncture of a cavity is termed

A. otony
B. centesis
C. ectomy
D. ostomy

29. When the patient is being transferred from the OR table after surgery, the action should be

A. swift but cautious in order to get the patient to the recovery room as quickly as possible
B. performed with comfort of the patient as the prime concern
C. gentle and rapid so that the patient does not wake up
D. gentle and slow in order to prevent circulatory depression

30. In steam sterilization, the function of pressure is to

A. destroy microorganisms
B. increase the temperature of the steam
C. lower the exposure time
D. create condensation

31. Which of the following suture materials is *not* generally used in the presence of infection?

A. silk
B. surgical gut
C. polypropylene
D. stainless steel

32. Radical surgery done for lower sigmoid or rectal malignancy is a/an

A. Wertheim's procedure
B. abdominal perineal resection
C. Whipple procedure
D. pelvic exenteration

33. The term for fluid or water in the ventricles of the brain is

A. hydrophobia
B. hydrocephalus
C. hydrocele
D. hydronephrosis

34. The patient may be left on the transport stretcher unattended

A. under no circumstances
B. if he or she is alert and responsible
C. if he or she is sound asleep
D. if he or she can be observed by passing personnel

35. 212° Farenheit is equivalent to

A. 32° centigrade
B. 98.6° centigrade
C. 100° centigrade
D. 175° centigrade

36. Bakes common duct dilators are available in sizes

A. 1–9
B. 5–13
C. 3–11
D. 3–13

37. A congenital abnormality of the musculature between the stomach and the duodenum is called

A. esophageal atresia
B. pyloric stenosis
C. intestinal atresia
D. duodenal atresia

38. Oblique means

A. up and down
B. side to side
C. right angle
D. slanting, diagonal

39. A procedure performed to treat myasthenia gravis is a/an

A. adrenalectomy
B. splenectomy
C. thymectomy
D. parathyroidectomy

40. In the steam sterilization process, only freshly laundered linen is used in order to

A. ensure sterilization
B. increase superheating
C. kill bacteria
D. decrease superheating

41. Following completion of colon anastomosis, the divided mesentery is closed with chromic suture to prevent

A. paralytic ileus
B. postoperative obstruction
C. postoperative hemorrhage
D. tissue necrosis

42. A forceps used to grasp lung tissue is a/an

A. Crile
B. Adson
C. Duval
D. Walton

43. The qualities of alcohol are

A. germicidal, tuberculocidal
B. germicidal, sporicidal
C. disinfectant, detergent
D. sterilant, sporicidal

44. A patient may be transported to the OR in a wheelchair if

A. there are no stretchers available
B. the patient is a child
C. the patient is not medicated
D. the patient's leg is in a cast

45. Ischemia can be defined as

A. excessive blood supply to a part
B. deficient blood supply to a part
C. abnormal condition of the hipbone
D. abnormal condition of the ischium and the anus

46. The person transporting the patient on a stretcher should

A. push the stretcher from the head
B. pull the stretcher by the foot
C. guide the stretcher from either side
D. guide the stretcher from any position that is comfortable

47. Activated glutaraldehyde

A. is corrosive to instruments
B. causes damage to lenses or the cement on lensed instruments
C. is absorbed by rubber and plastic
D. can be reused

48. A Gelpi is a

A. dissector
B. grasper
C. hemostat
D. retractor

49. Digestion of pancreatic tissue by the exocrines that it secretes is known clinically as

A. pancreatic cyst
B. pseudocyst
C. pancreatitis
D. steatorrhea

50. Deflation of pneumoperitoneum after trocar removal is prevented by the presence on the outer cannula of a

A. stopcock
B. sealing cap
C. piston valve
D. needle guard

51. A tiny tubular tract that may have a skin opening beside the anus and that carries into the anal canal is called a/an

A. fissure in ano
B. fistula in ano
C. ischiorectal abscess
D. hemorrhoid

52. The word arthrodesis means

A. reconstruction of a joint
B. fracture of a joint
C. immobilization of a joint
D. reduction of a joint

53. What method of sterilization is used for liquids?

A. slow exhaust
B. fast exhaust
C. gas
D. dry heat

54. Medullary canal reamers are used to insert

A. Smith Petersen nails
B. Richards nails
C. Jewett nails
D. Küntscher nails

55. A protrusion of fat through an abdominal wall defect between the xyphoid process and umbilicus is a/an

A. umbilical hernia
B. diaphragmatic hernia
C. epigastric hernia
D. Spigelian hernia

56. The position frequently utilized in thyroid and gallbladder surgery is

A. supine
B. Trendelenburg
C. reverse Trendelenburg
D. dorsal recumbent

57. What part of the cell is destroyed in steam sterilization?

A. cell protein
B. ovum
C. monocyte
D. basophil

58. Which scope has a trocar?

A. cystoscope
B. laparoscope
C. laryngoscope
D. bronchoscope

59. Bowel decompression intraoperatively is maintained by use of a/an

A. antispasmodic medication
B. warm packs
C. nasogastric tube
D. rectal tube

60. A rotator cuff tear would occur in the

A. hip
B. shoulder
C. ankle
D. knee

61. Which position would be chosen for a pneumonectomy?

A. supine
B. dorsal
C. lateral
D. Kraske

62. When preparing tubing or any item with a lumen for gas sterilization,

A. a residual of distilled water should be left in the lumen
B. the lumen should be blown out with air to force-dry before packaging
C. a residual of saline should be left in the lumen
D. it does not matter if it is moist or dry

63. A rib raspatory is a

A. Sauerbruck
B. Alexander
C. Josephs
D. Stille-Luer

64. A right-angled gallbladder forceps is a

A. Crile
B. mixter
C. Jackson
D. Rochester-Pean

65. A self-retaining mouth gag with assorted blades is a

A. Jennings
B. Dingman
C. Castro
D. Cushing

66. The storage life for a muslin-wrapped item on open shelving is

A. 7 days or less
B. 14 days or less
C. 21 days or less
D. 30 days or less

67. How are the legs placed in the lateral position?

A. both legs are straight
B. both legs are flexed
C. the lower leg is flexed, the upper leg straight
D. the lower leg is straight, the upper leg flexed

68. Which gland plays a role in the immune mechanism of the body?

A. thymus
B. pineal
C. hypothalamus
D. adrenals

69. The islets of Langerhans manufacture

A. insulin
B. adrenaline
C. ACTH
D. epinephrine

70. Which nerve travels down the back side of the thigh?

A. sciatic
B. gluteal
C. peroneal
D. pudendal

71. When moving a patient from lithotomy position,

A. lower legs together quickly
B. lower legs together slowly
C. lower each leg separately and slowly
D. lower each leg separately and quickly

72. If a sterile package drops to the floor

A. it should never be used
B. it may be used if it is paper wrapped
C. it may be used if the floor is dry
D. it may be used if it is dusted off

73. A tonsil suction is a

A. Young
B. Poole
C. Frazier
D. Yankauer

74. In a cholydochotomy the common bile duct is

A. aspirated
B. removed
C. explored
D. x-rayed

75. The principal hazard encountered in splenectomy is

A. trauma to adjacent structures
B. hypertension
C. hemorrhage
D. poor visualization of organs

76. The serosal intestinal layer is usually closed with

A. continuous silk suture
B. interrupted silk suture
C. continuous chromic suture
D. interrupted chromic suture

77. An item used to force blood from an extremity when a tourniquet is being used is a/an

A. stockingette
B. tourniquet cuff
C. Robert Jones bandage
D. Esmarch bandage

78. Which is an acceptable means of pouring a sterile solution onto a sterile field?

A. the scrub nurse holds a receptacle away from the table as the circulator pours
B. the scrub nurse sets the receptable near the edge of a waterproof-draped table
C. all solutions are poured over the ring stand by the circulator
D. A and B

79. What nerve is affected by pressure on the lower leg or knee?

A. phrenic
B. pudendal
C. perineal
D. peroneal

80. The thyroid, cricoid, and epiglottic cartilages are located in the

A. larynx
B. pharynx
C. trachea
D. hyoid

81. The structure that covers the entrance of the larynx when one swallows, thus preventing food from entering the airway (trachea) is called

A. glottis
B. vocal fold
C. epiglottis
D. oropharynx

82. Which paired set of bones unite to form the upper jawbone?

A. frontal
B. maxillary
C. ethmoid
D. sphenoid

83. In the lateral chest position, a sandbag or padding is placed under the chest at axillary level to

A. facilitate respiration
B. aid in position stability
C. prevent pressure on the lower arm
D. create good body alignment

84. A ventilation system that provides a rapid air exchange in a unidirectional flow is called

A. turbulence control flow
B. conventional fresh air flow
C. conventional filtered air recirculation
D. laminar flow

85. Which of the following is frequently used over an incision in pediatric surgery?

A. collodian
B. benzoin
C. pressure dressing
D. cotton-elastic bandage

86. Choledochostomy is drained by means of a

A. Penrose drain
B. sump drain
C. T tube
D. cholangiocath

87. The instrument used to measure the depth of the uterus during a dilation and curettage is a

A. Sim's curette
B. Jacob's forceps
C. Boseman forceps
D. uterine sound

88. Vagotomy is performed for peptic ulcer disease to

A. decrease transmission of pain stimuli
B. increase secretion of gastrin
C. increase circulation to the greater curvature
D. decrease secretion of gastric acid

89. Before surgery, elastic bandages are sometimes applied to the lower extremities to

A. prevent pressure areas
B. prevent skin irritation
C. prevent embolus formation
D. keep the legs warm

90. Surgical masks should be changed

A. after each case
B. daily
C. twice a day
D. every 2 hours

91. Why would benzoin be applied to the skin before dressing application?

A. to facilitate easier removal
B. to increase adhesiveness
C. to add a microbial film to the skin
D. to prevent allergic reaction to tape

92. Closing the internal os of an incompetent cervix with a ligature of tape is called

A. Manchester
B. Wertheim
C. Shirodkar
D. Le Fort

93. Pneumoperitoneum is effected by instilling gas into the peritoneal cavity by way of a

A. Silverman needle
B. Verres needle
C. trocar
D. Craig needle

94. In addition to providing bladder drainage following a suprapubic prostatectomy, a Foley catheter

A. exerts pressure to obtain hemostasis
B. provides for bladder expansion
C. prevents nosocomial infection
D. prevents bladder atrophy

95. Electrical connection of the patient to the conductive floor is assured by

A. a conductive strap over the sheet covering the patient
B. a conductive table mattress
C. a conductive strap in direct contact with the patient's skin, with one end of the strap fastened to the OR table metal frame
D. a ground plate under the patient

96. Countershock is used

A. after all CPR efforts have proved unsuccessful

B. when ventricular fibrillation or ventricular tachycardia without pulse is evident
C. if the pulse cannot be restored
D. once the airway is opened

97. The heavy bone that extends from the scapula to the elbow is the

A. radius
B. ulna
C. humerus
D. tibia

98. Skeletal muscle is

A. voluntary, smooth
B. involuntary, smooth
C. voluntary, striated
D. involuntary, striated

99. Which structure attaches bones to muscles?

A. ligament
B. aponeurosis
C. tendon
D. fascia

100. The following are all contraindications to vaginal hysterectomy *except*

A. a large uterus
B. malignancy
C. adnexal mass
D. presence of a cystocele

101. Instruments used to close the vaginal vault in an abdominal hysterectomy must be

A. kept separate from the setup before use
B. considered contaminated after use
C. noncrushing clamps
D. kept on the Mayo stand after use

102. Another name for scapulae is

A. shoulder blades
B. collar bones
C. corocoid process
D. acromian process

103. The Scarpa fascia would be encountered in surgery for a

A. gallbladder
B. spleen
C. hernia
D. thyroid

104. How many lobes are there in the left lung?

A. one
B. two
C. three
D. four

105. A constant closed suction that utilizes a plastic container serving as both a suction and a receptacle for blood is a

A. Hemovac
B. Robinson
C. Sengstaken-Blakemore
D. Potts-Smith

106. The medullary cavity is filled with

A. ossein
B. osteoblasts
C. red bone marrow
D. yellow bone marrow

107. Syphilis is caused by

A. herpes simplex
B. *Neisseria gonorrhoeae*
C. trichomoniasis
D. *Treponema pallidum*

108. A dye used in urinary diagnostic procedures is

A. methylene blue
B. fluorescein
C. gentian violet
D. anilene

109. Which stage of wound healing takes place in an aseptic wound with minimum tissue destruction and tissue reaction?

A. first (primary)
B. second (granulation)
C. third (delayed)
D. fourth (danger)

110. An abnormal accumulation of fluid in the tunica vaginalis is referred to as a

A. cystocele
B. hydrocele
C. spermatocele
D. varicocele

111. Periosteum is lifted from the surface of the bone with a/an

A. rongeur
B. curette
C. osteotome
D. elevator

112. Repair of a cranial defect is surgically represented by the term

A. trephination
B. cranioplasty
C. craniosynostosis
D. craniectomy

113. The cruciate ligament is located in the

A. knee
B. ankle
C. shoulder
D. elbow

114. Which organ contains the islets of Langerhans?

A. stomach
B. heart
C. liver
D. pancreas

115. When suprapubic drainage is in place the patient is

A. unable to void
B. able to void if the tube is unclamped
C. encouraged to void while the tube is clamped
D. less likely to void as quickly as he would with a urethral catheter

116. An ohmmeter tests

A. air humidity
B. conductivity
C. air temperature
D. explosibility

117. What is the purpose of a chest tube and water-seal drainage?

A. evacuate fluid and air
B. evacuate lung secretions
C. oxygenate the lung
D. plug the hole in the chest wall

118. Extreme flexion of the thighs in the lithotomy position impairs

A. circulatory function
B. respiratory function
C. nerve continuity
D. operative ability

119. A femoral-popliteal bypass is scheduled. Which self-retaining retractor would be used to facilitate exploration of the femoral artery?

A. Mason-Judd
B. DeBakey
C. Weitlaner
D. Gelpi

120. A double-bowl-shaped glass evacuator used to irrigate the bladder during transurethral surgery is called a/an

A. Robb
B. Valentine
C. Ellik
D. Toomey

121. Surgical interruption of selected posterior spinal nerve roots between the ganglion and the cord is called

A. laminectomy
B. rhizotomy
C. thermocoagulation
D. cordotomy

122. The structure(s) whose secretion is released in response to sexual stimulation is (are) the

A. seminal vesicle
B. ejaculatory duct
C. bulbourethral glands
D. prostate gland

123. In which intention of healing is there a wide, fibrous scar?

A. primary
B. secondary
C. third
D. fourth

124. Which bacteria cause many boils, carbuncles, and internal abscesses?

A. *Escherichia coli*
B. *Salmonella*
C. *Clostridium perfringens*
D. *Staphylococcus aureus*

125. An osmotic diuretic agent used in neurosurgery to reduce cerebral edema is

A. Lasix
B. mannitol
C. Diamox
D. ammonium chloride

126. Which structure joins the clavicle medially?

A. scapula
B. sternum
C. humerus
D. acromioclavicular joint

127. What is the reason for using cortisone?

A. anti-inflammatory
B. antibacterial
C. antihistamine
D. antisuppressant

128. Hemorrhage is suspected if

A. the blood pressure drops in direct relationship to the drop in the pulse
B. the blood pressure drops and pulse rate rises
C. there is no change in the blood pressure, only in the pulse rate
D. the blood pressure elevates and the pulse drops

129. How many feet above the ground is considered safe for electrical outlets and fixtures that are not explosion-proof?

A. 1
B. 3
C. 5
D. 7

130. Carpal tunnel syndrome affects the

A. elbow
B. hand
C. knee
D. ankle

131. An abnormal whitening of mucous membrane considered to be a precancerous lesion is termed

A. hemangioma
B. glossitis
C. leukoplakia
D. leukorrhea

132. When the foreskin of the penis cannot be retracted over the glans it is called

A. hypospadias
B. ptosis
C. phimosis
D. balanitis

133. The burn characterized by blister formation, pain, and a moist and mottled red appearance is

A. first
B. second
C. third
D. fourth

134. Microorganisms whose growth is inhibited by free oxygen are

A. spores
B. aerobes
C. faculative bacteria
D. anaerobes

135. Sperm are produced in _____ and are stored in the _____

A. the testes, vas deferens
B. the prostate gland, testes
C. Cowper's gland, vas deferens
D. the vas deferens, testes

136. The part of the eye that receives images and transmits them to the brain is the

A. retina
B. lens
C. choroid
D. cornea

137. The term idiopathic when referring to disease means

A. disease producing
B. known cause
C. undetermined cause
D. new growth of cells

138. Drugs used to contract the uterus after delivery of the placenta are called

A. glycosides
B. oxytocics
C. hormones
D. antispasmodics

139. Which of the following instruments would be used to retract the bladder walls during a suprapubic prostatectomy?

A. Weitlaner
B. O'Sullivan-O'Conner
C. Mason-Judd
D. Dennis-Brown

140. Maintenance of bony exposure during a lumbar laminectomy is effected by the use of a

A. Gelpi
B. Finochietto
C. Cloward
D. Beckman-Adson

141. A common abdominal complication caused by repeated pelvic inflammatory disease is

A. adenomyosis
B. endometriosis
C. adhesions
D. vaginal discharge

142. Which of the following shunts would be used surgically to correct hydrocephalus?

A. Scribner

B. Brisman-Nova
C. Le Veen
D. Hakim

143. A spinal fusion is usually effected by autogenous grafts taken from the patient's

A. ischium
B. ileum
C. ilium
D. lamina

144. A lateral deviation in the position of the great toe is termed

A. Dupuytren's contracture
B. hallux valgus
C. spondylitis
D. Volkmann's contracture

145. The transparent anatomic structure known as the "window of the eye" is the

A. sclera
B. ciliary body
C. cornea
D. lens

146. Epinephrine, which prepares the body to meet emergency situations, is secreted by

A. pituitary gland
B. pancreas
C. thymus
D. adrenal gland

147. Nosocomial infection refers to

A. hospital-acquired infection
B. infection in the nose
C. infection in the wound
D. surgery-related infection

148. Hand placement for cardiac compression during CPR is

A. heel of hand over the xiphoid process, heel of other hand on top of it
B. heel of hand over lower third of sternum (above xiphoid process), other hand on top of it
C. fingertips over lower third of sternum, other hand on top of back of hand
D. heel of hand over heart area, other hand on top of it

149. The edges of a wrapper that enclose sterile contents are considered

A. sterile
B. semi-sterile
C. unsterile
D. surgically clean

150. A ureteral stent catheter is used to

A. remove ureteral calculi
B. inject dye through in pyelography
C. provide long-term drainage in ureteral obstruction
D. provide a ureteral marker

151. Colpocleisis is a

A. Manchester procedure
B. Wertheim procedure
C. Le Fort procedure
D. Rubin's test

152. A condition characterized by excruciating, piercing pain in the face is known as

A. Meniere's disease
B. acoustic neuritis
C. tic douloureux
D. tinnitis

153. Which of the following instruments is *not* found in a vaginal procedure?

A. Goodell dilator
B. Jacobs tenaculum
C. Auvard speculum
D. Harrington retractor

154. The operation to correct prolapse of the anterior vaginal wall is

A. colporrhapy
B. Shirodkar
C. Le Fort
D. vesicourethral suspension

155. Which nasal sinus can be approached *only* through an external eyebrow incision?

A. sphenoid
B. ethmoid
C. frontal
D. maxillary

156. Which sinus is surgically opened in a Caldwell-Luc procedure?

A. ethmoid
B. frontal
C. maxillary
D. sphenoid

157. Which of the following pieces of hardware will be used in an intramedullary fixation of a fracture of an adult femoral shaft?

A. Kirschner wire
B. Steinmann pin
C. Küntscher nail
D. Jewett nail

158. The tenth cranial nerve is the

A. oculomotor
B. trigeminal
C. acoustic
D. vagus

159. The normal body temperature in centigrade measurement is

A. 37°C
B. 56°C
C. 98°C
D. 112°C

160. Once the skin knife is used

A. discard it from the sterile setup
B. place it in a specimen basin
C. remove the blade from the handle and discard the blade
D. place it on the back table

161. Which tube is used for gastrointestinal decompression?

A. Penrose
B. Poole
C. Ferguson
D. Levin

162. Complete displacement of one articular surface of a joint from another is called a/an

A. subluxation
B. dislocation
C. avulsion
D. epiphyseal separation

163. Continuous irrigation of the bladder is necessary during cystoscopy to

A. keep the area moistened and thus reduce trauma
B. distend the bladder walls for visualization
C. act as a viewing medium
D. reduce heat from the lighted scope

164. The excision and removal of diseased and necrotic tissue is termed

A. desiccation
B. degloving
C. debridement
D. dermabrasion

165. The excision of loose skin and periorbital fat of the eyelids is called

A. fasciectomy
B. oculoplasty
C. rhytidectomy
D. blepharoplasty

166. A fleshy encroachment onto the cornea is called

A. chalazion
B. glaucoma
C. pterygium
D. strabismus

167. The hormone-releasing center of the brain is the

A. hypothalamus
B. medulla
C. pons
D. brainstem

168. The olecranon process is located at the

A. shoulder
B. knee
C. ankle
D. elbow

169. What is the ovarian follicle?

A. ova and their surrounding tissue in varying stages of development
B. deep ovarian connective tissue
C. endocrine gland containing mature ovum
D. product of ovulation

170. Which ligaments attach the uterus to either side of the pelvic cavity?

A. uterosacral
B. cardinal
C. broad
D. rectouterine

171. Carbohydrates are the basic source of

A. energy
B. oxygen
C. growth
D. repair of tissue

172. Bradycardia is

A. heartbeat over 100 beats per minute
B. irregular heartbeat
C. thready, weak heartbeat
D. heartbeat less than 60 beats per minute

173. If a needle punctures a sterile team member's glove,

A. discard the needle
B. change the glove
C. place another glove over the punctured one
D. A and B

174. Which type of laser emission is heavily absorbed by water?

A. argon

B. Nd-YAG
C. CO_2
D. FEL

175. Progesterone is secreted by the

A. graafian follicle
B. pituitary gland
C. corpus luteum
D. thyroid gland

176. Surgical treatment that reduces intraocular pressure by releasing the aqueous fluids into the subconjunctival tissues is called

A. iridectomy
B. cyclodiathermy
C. iridencleisis
D. cyclodialysis

177. An instrument used to incise the eardrum to relieve pressure is called a

A. Rosen knife
B. Walsh crurotomy knife
C. myringotomy knife
D. Hough pick

178. In which surgical specialty would a perfusionist be necessary?

A. neurologic surgery
B. cardiovascular surgery
C. transplant surgery
D. microsurgery

179. The preferred method of gloving is _____. In changing during a case, this method _____ be used.

A. closed, can
B. open, can
C. open, cannot
D. closed, cannot

180. Respirations increase during

A. shock
B. poisoning
C. diabetic coma
D. fever

181. An infected wound left open to heal on its own without sutures heals

A. first
B. second
C. third
D. fourth

182. The malleus, incus, and stapes are located in the

A. middle ear
B. outer ear
C. inner ear
D. external ear

183. The temperature taken rectally is

A. the same as the temperature taken orally
B. about 1.0°F above the temperature taken orally
C. about 1.0°F below the temperature taken orally
D. the same as the temperature taken in the axilla

184. When gloving a surgeon,

A. keep the palm of the glove facing the surgeon
B. avoid contact by keeping your thumbs tucked in
C. hold the second glove while doing the first
D. glove only over a sterile area

185. Ringing in the ears is known as

A. tympanitis
B. tinnitus
C. presbycusis
D. vertigo

186. A device that produces an intense, coherent, directional beam of light by stimulated electronic or molecular transitions to a lower energy level is a/an

A. cryoprove
B. fiberoptic unit
C. laser
D. electrocautery unit

187. If the patient has a positive breast biopsy and the surgeon proceeds to do a radical mastectomy,

A. the same drapes and instruments may be used
B. the patient is reprepped, and new drapes and instruments are used
C. the drapes may remain but new instruments are used
D. the drapes are replaced but the same instruments may be used

188. At which artery is the blood pressure taken?

A. cephalic
B. brachial
C. basilar
D. axillary

189. The action of white blood cells is to

A. transport oxygen
B. clot blood
C. produce enzymes
D. destroy bacteria

190. What is the function of the endocrine glands?

A. manufacture sugar
B. produce hormones
C. maintain acid-base balance
D. digest fat

191. Oxygenated blood is carried to the heart via

A. pulmonary artery
B. pulmonary vein
C. carotid artery
D. carotid vein

192. Where is bile produced?

A. gallbladder
B. liver
C. duodenum
D. hepatic duct

193. Which nerve is compressed in the carpal canal as a result of carpal tunnel syndrome?

A. brachial
B. radial
C. median
D. ulnar

194. Endoscopic secretions or washings for laboratory study must be collected in a/an

A. suction pump
B. emesis basin
C. Lukens trap
D. McCarthy evacuator

195. During vascular surgery an arteriotomy is executed with a #11 blade and extended by use of a

A. Lahey
B. Metzenbaum
C. Potts-Smith
D. Stevens

196. What is an evisceration?

A. partial or total splitting open of a wound
B. separation of the layers of a wound
C. protrusion of viscera through an abdominal incision
D. failure of a wound to heal evenly

197. The first part of the small intestine is known as the

A. jejunum
B. pylorus
C. duodenum
D. ileum

198. What organisms are likely to be found in a surgical wound adjacent to colostomy?

A. *Staphylococcus*
B. *Streptococcus*
C. *Pseudomonas*
D. *Escherichia coli*

199. A liter would be the equivalent to

A. 250 ml (cc)
B. 500 ml (cc)
C. 750 ml (cc)
D. 1000 ml (cc)

200. When inserting a Foley catheter, always

A. check the integrity of the bag by inflating it with the correct amount of sterile water prior to insertion
B. inflate the bag immediately after insertion
C. connect the catheter to the closed drainage system before the catheter is inserted
D. have the scrub nurse hold bag above table level

201. The proper setting for a tourniquet applied to the leg is

A. 100–200 mm Hg
B. 250–300 mm Hg
C. 350–400 mm Hg
D. 400–500 mm Hg

202. Crushing a urinary calculus in the bladder through the urethra is called

A. cystolithotomy
B. litholapaxy
C. urethrotomy
D. urethroplasty

203. The surgical procedure performed for recurrent acute epididymitis is

A. epididymectomy
B. orchiectomy
C. vasectomy
D. orchiopexy

204. When doing an abdominal prep, the umbilicus is

A. done first
B. done last or separately
C. given no special consideration
D. avoided because it is contaminated

205. The portion of the stomach located at the approach to the small intestine is the

A. cardia
B. fundus
C. pylorus
D. antrum

206. What is the action of Lasix?

A. anti-inflammatory
B. diuretic
C. depressant (CNS)
D. contrast media

207. The normal bladder capacity is

A. 100–200 ml
B. 200–300 ml
C. 700–800 ml
D. 800–1000 ml

208. Rectal surgery preparation is done

A. top to bottom
B. bottom to top
C. surrounding area first, anus last
D. anus first, surrounding area last

209. When changing a gown during a case, the _____ is(are) removed first, the _____ second, and a rescrub is _____.

A. gown, gloves, not necessary
B. gloves, gown, not necessary
C. gown, gloves, necessary
D. gloves, gown, necessary

210. Which piece of equipment is used to make a skin graft larger?

A. knife dermatome
B. Brown air dermatome
C. skin mesher dermatome
D. Reese drum-type dermatome

211. The majority of calculi in the urinary tract are composed of

A. calcium
B. uric acid
C. cystine
D. mixed elements

212. In which structure is urine collected before passing down the ureters into the bladder?

A. renal pelvis
B. calyces
C. Bowman's capsule
D. collecting tubules

213. The kidneys are held in place by the

A. renal columns
B. detrusor muscle
C. renal fascia and fat
D. tunica fibrosa

214. A culture and sensitivity is done to

A. determine nature of organism and the susceptibility of that organism
B. diagnose blood infections
C. culture a single organism responsible for infection
D. determine if furniture and rooms are being cleaned properly

215. Which of the following is considered the *most* effective agent for scrubbing?

A. povidone-iodine
B. glutaraldehyde
C. hexachlorophene
D. chlorhexidene

216. All of the following would be on the setup for an open thoracotomy *except*

A. Alexander's periosteotome
B. Langenbeck elevator
C. Joseph's saw
D. Lebsche knife

217. The term used to signify that a specific fracture has not healed in the time considered average for that fracture is

A. nonunion
B. delayed union
C. malunion
D. ossification

218. During a basic femoral head fixation, the first piece of hardware utilized is a/an

A. guide wire
B. compression screw
C. hip nail
D. intertrochanteric plate

219. The hormone produced in the ovaries, responsible for the development and maintenance of most female secondary sex characteristics is

A. leutinizing hormone
B. testosterone
C. adrenocorticotropin
D. estrogen

220. The funnel-shaped, open end of each fallopian tube is called the

A. infundibulum
B. fimbriae
C. tunica albuginea
D. stroma

221. When doing a skin prep on a patient with a stoma, the stoma is

A. done first because it is open
B. done last or separately
C. given no special consideration
D. avoided since it is contaminated

222. Why would a patient come to the OR wearing elastic stockings?

A. to supply warmth
B. to prevent thrombus formation
C. to increase cardiac function
D. to decrease blood flow to legs

223. The purpose of the surgical hand scrub is to render the skin

A. sterile
B. surgically clean
C. disinfected
D. aseptic

224. The gas introduced into the peritoneum during laparoscopy to create a pneumoperitoneum is

A. nitrous oxide
B. oxygen
C. nitrogen
D. carbon dioxide

225. Crutchfield tongs produce skeletal traction to reduce fractures of the

A. phalanges
B. femoral shaft
C. cervical spine
D. humeral shaft

226. Which disease could be transmitted via a blood transfusion?

A. hepatitis A
B. hepatitis B
C. infectious hepatitis
D. hepatonephritis

227. *Staphylococcus* is usually transmitted by

A. sexual contact
B. upper respiratory tract
C. urine
D. feces

228. A bacteria with a thick coat which protects it from temperature extremes or strong chemicals is a

A. parasite
B. host
C. saprophyte
D. spore

229. When a three-way Foley catheter is used, the third lumen is for

A. drainage
B. balloon inflation
C. continuous irrigation
D. constant suction

230. If a towel clip must be removed during a procedure,

A. the patient must be redraped
B. discard it from the field and cover the area with another sterile drape
C. place it near the skin knife
D. use the same towel clip but cover the area with another sterile drape

231. A retractor used to maintain subluxation of the femoral head in a total hip replacement is a

A. Hohmann
B. Bennett
C. Hibbs
D. Richardson

232. Why would a *Pseudomonas* organism take up residence in a burned area of body?

A. skin no longer an effective barrier
B. interrupted blood supply
C. depression of immune system
D. inflammatory response

233. Which specimen would be placed in formalin?

A. bronchial washings
B. tonsils
C. breast biopsy/frozen
D. kidney stones

234. A legal wrong committed by one person involving injury to another person is called a/an

A. tort
B. default
C. liability
D. impressment

235. Scoliosis is surgically treated by the implantation of

A. Steinmann pins
B. Rush rods
C. Lottes nails
D. Harrington rods

236. An intravenous agent used for anesthesia induction is

A. lidocaine
B. Fluothane
C. Pentothal sodium
D. Demerol

237. When using a hyperthermia blanket, the heating fluid must be maintained constantly and not allowed to exceed

A. 18°C
B. 25°C
C. 35°C
D. 42°C

238. Unauthorized discussion of a patient's surgery outside of the OR constitutes a lawsuit for

A. defamation
B. negligence
C. assault and battery
D. invasion of privacy

239. When applying a sterile sheet on the patient,

A. protect the gloved hands by cuffing the end of the sheet over them
B. adjust the drape by pulling it towards the sterile area
C. the gloved hands may touch the painted skin of the patient
D. unfold from the patient's foot to the operative site

240. A chronic granulomatous inflammation of a Meibomian gland in the eyelid is a/an

A. entropion
B. chalazion
C. blepharochalasis
D. pterygium

241. Which of the following is a barbiturate given for its hypnotic effect preoperatively?

A. anectine
B. Demerol
C. atropine
D. secobarbital (Seconal)

242. When is bowel technique necessary?

A. when a case is considered septic
B. when the patient has not had a bowel prep
C. when the patient has perforated preoperatively
D. when a contaminated area of the intestinal tract is entered

243. A slowly progressive contracture of the palmar fascia is called

A. Volkmann's contracture
B. carpal tunnel syndrome
C. Dupuytren's contracture
D. talipes valgus

244. If rubber suction tubing is to be reused,

  A. the lumen must be flushed with a detergent-disinfectant before tubing is terminally sterilized

  B. it must be cold-sterilized between uses

  C. it requires no special procedure

  D. the lumen must be flushed with water and sterilized

245. If the scrub nurse receives a broken needle back from the surgeon, she should

  A. report it to the circulator

  B. report it to the supervisor

  C. tell the surgeon immediately

  D. make a mental note until the final count

246. Heparin is a/an

  A. reagent

  B. anticoagulant

  C. coagulant

  D. neutralizing agent

247. Neo-Synephrine

  A. constricts blood vessels

  B. dilates blood vessels

  C. constricts pupil

  D. dilates pupil

248. The legal doctrine *Res ipsa Loquitor* applies to

  A. invasion of privacy

  B. an employer's liability for an employee's negligence

  C. accountability

  D. injuries sustained by the patient in the OR due to negligence

249. After a case is completed, the sterile team members

  A. discard gown and gloves before leaving the OR suite

  B. discard gown and keep gloves on to transport soiled equipment

  C. discard gown, gloves, caps, masks, and shoe covers before leaving OR suite

  D. discard gown, gloves, and masks before the room is dismantled

250. Pilocarpine is used to

  A. dilate the pupil

  B. constrict the pupil

  C. keep the eye moist

  D. reduce inflammation

Answers and Explanations

1. **(B)** When an inguinal herniorrhaphy is being performed the spermatic cord is identified, freed, and a Penrose drain is placed around it for traction, and to prevent injury. *(17:238)*

2. **(B)** Polyglycolic acid is a synthetic absorbable suture which is not affected by enzymes but rather by the process of hydrolysis, whereby water in the body acts to break down the polymeric constituents. *(35:14)*

3. **(D)** Twenty-seven pounds of pressure is necessary for the steam autoclave set at 270°F. The high speed is the flash sterilizer. *(32:57)*

4. **(A)** The leukocytes (white blood cells) normally range between 5,000 and 10,000 cells in each cu mm of whole blood. High white counts may be indicative of an unsuspected inflammatory process which could contraindicate surgery. It would not be contraindicated if surgery were to treat an infectious condition, e.g., acute appendicitis. *(7:653; 25:53)*

5. **(C)** The suffix *itis* means inflammation. Appendicitis is an inflammation of the appendix. Tracheitis is an inflammation of the trachea. *(36:883)*

6. **(C)** Meckel's diverticulum is a congenital sac or blind pouch sometimes found in the lower portion of the ileum. Strangulation may cause an intestinal obstruction. *(36:1015)*

7. **(C)** When a Frazier suction is used, a stylette must accompany it in order to clear the suction if it becomes clogged. *(32:727)*

8. **(D)** Recirculation of filtered air at a rate of no less than 25 air exchanges per hour is considered safe and economical. *(2:83)*

9. **(A)** Derogatory statements made about one person to another is defamation. In writing it is libel. If oral, it is slander. *(17:416)*

10. **(D)** This symbol in Latin means without: sine (s̄). *(36:1933)*

11. **(B)** Telephone, telegram, or written permission is acceptable. If by phone two people monitor conversation and sign permission form as witnesses. *(2:45)*

12. **(A)** Instruments completely unwrapped sterilize at 3 minutes. The autoclave is set at 270°F. *(2:99)*

13. **(A)** The tissue through which retention sutures are passed includes the skin, subcutaneous tissue, fascia, and may include the rectus muscle and peritoneum of an abdominal incision. *(2:263)*

14. **(B)** Indirect hernias leave the abdominal cavity through the inguinal canal. Consequently the hernia can often be found in the scrotum. *(32:153)*

15. **(B)** Dead space is that space caused by separation of wound edges that have not been closely approximated by sutures. *(2:239)*

16. **(C)** Unwrapped tubing is autoclaved at 270°F for a minimum of 10 minutes. A residual of distilled water should be left in the lumen. *(2:95, 99)*

17. **(D)** Some diabetic, geriatric, and also patients who have varicosities who are prone to embolus formation or have a history of embolus, wear antiembolic stockings or elastic bandages on the lower extremities to prevent embolic phenomena. *(2:62, 63, 66)*

18. **(B)** Hypovolemia means low or decreased blood volume. *Hypo* means below. *Volemia* refers to blood volume. *(2:162)*

19. **(D)** An angiogram is a test in which vessel size, location, and configuration can be studied by injecting dye into intracranial vessels. It is an x-ray procedure. An angiogram can be done of the aorta, heart, and brain. *(32:719)*

20. **(C)** Instruments alone can be flashed at 270°F. The addition of rubber tube makes the requirement 10 minutes at 270°F. *(2:99)*

21. **(A)** Nonabsorbable sutures remain permanently embedded in the body. During the healing process, they become encapsulated with fibrous tissue. *(35:74)*

22. **(B)** This procedure is performed to remove a malignant lesion of the right colon and in some cases to remove inflammatory lesions involving the ileum, cecum, or right colon (ascending colon). *(32:229)*

23. **(B)** Adduction is movement toward the median plane. This is a vertical plane through the trunk and head dividing the body into right and left halves. Abduction means movement away from the median plane. *(36:5, 36, 1016)*

24. **(B)** Drainage tubing should be placed so that there is a downward gravity flow. The drainage bag should be below the level of the tubing. This prevents retrograde flow which could contaminate the bladder. *(2:150)*

25. **(C)** Linen packs must not exceed a maximum size of 12 × 12 × 20 inches. Linens are loosely criss-crossed so as not to form a dense mass. *(2:95)*

26. **(B)** A retention or stay suture provides a secondary suture line. The purpose is to relieve undue strain on the primary suture line and to help obliterate dead space. *(32:110)*

27. **(B)** After complete exposure of the biliary tract, the cystic artery is doubly ligated and divided. The cystic duct is identified, carefully dissected from the common bile duct to the gallbladder neck, then doubly ligated and divided. *(32:187)*

28. **(B)** Centesis is a puncture of a cavity. Amniocentesis is a puncture of the amniotic sac. Thoracentesis is a puncture of the chest cavity. *(36:295)*

29. **(D)** The patient should be lifted or rolled gently and slowly to prevent circulatory depression. A sudden or jarring movement is potentially dangerous to the patient. *(2:149)*

30. **(B)** Moist heat and steam under pressure destroy microbial life. Heat destroys microorganisms but process is hastened with steam. Pressure is necessary to increase the temperature of the steam for destruction of microbial life. *(2:82)*

31. **(A)** Silk suture is used only in the absence of infection. For its use during the infectious process may cause granulomas and ultimate sinus formation. *(2:257)*

32. **(B)** This surgery is performed for malignant lesions of the lower sigmoid colon, rectum, and anus. It is a two-part procedure which involves resecting the proximal disease-free sigmoid and pulling the diseased portion down through a widely excised anus with total, permanent closure of the anus. *(32:232)*

33. **(B)** The increased accumulation of cerebrospinal fluid within the ventricles of the brain is hydrocephalus. It results from interference with normal circulation and absorption of fluid and may result from developmental anomalies, infection, injury, or brain tumors. Treatment may be a surgical shunt through which cerebrospinal fluid flows from the ventricles of the brain to a cavity such as the peritoneal. *(36:785)*

34. **(A)** A patient should never be left on a stretcher or OR table unattended, even though appearing alert and responsible. One of the major causes of litigation is injury resulting from an accident that occurred when a medicated patient was left unattended (abandoned). *(11:288)*

35. **(C)** The boiling point of water is 212°F. This is equal to 100°C.

$$1.0°F = 0.54°C$$

Formula

When you know	You can convert to	When you use
Degrees F	Degrees C	$5/9 \, (F-32) = C$
Degrees C	Degrees F	$9/5 \, (C) + 32 = F$

Example   212F
−32

$$180 \times 5/9 = 100$$

(36:218, 1905)

36. **(C)** Bakes common duct dilators are available in sizes 3–11. *(32:188)*

37. **(B)** Congenital hypertrophic pyloric stenosis is an abnormality of the pyloric musculature in which there is alteration of fibrous, gristle-like tissue, causing mechanical obstruction of the distal stomach. *(7:223)*

38. **(D)** Oblique means slanting or diagonal. An x-ray may be taken at an oblique angle. An incision such as a Kochers or one for an inguinal hernia are considered oblique. *(36:1150)*

39. **(C)** Removal of the non-neoplastic thymus gland appears to have equivocal effects on the progression of myasthenia gravis. There is, however, a statistical basis that the procedure has a high curative rate when done on females.   *(7:1238)*

40. **(D)** Linen must be laundered to rehydrate between sterilization exposures to ensure sufficient moisture content of the fibers. This prevents superheating thus absorption of the sterilizing agent (steam) which could alter microbial destruction.   *(2:97; 32:53)*

41. **(B)** Surgical closure of the mesenteric defect is of paramount importance. A loop of intestines may become trapped postoperatively and result in postoperative intestinal obstruction.   *(11:187)*

42. **(C)** The Duval lung-grasping forceps is designed to grasp lung tissue firmly while producing minimal tissue trauma.   *(6:232)*

43. **(A)** Alcohol is an active germicide against tubercle bacilli in concentrations of 70 to 90%. It is not superficial. It is more useful as an antiseptic than as a disinfectant.   *(32:64)*

44. **(C)** Wheelchairs are not considered a safe method of transporting medicated patients but are an acceptable method for nonmedicated patients. It is the nurse's responsibility to protect the patient.   *(5:23)*

45. **(B)** From the Greek *ischeim* meaning to hold back, plus *haima* meaning blood. Local or temporary deficiency of blood supply due to obstruction of the circulation to a part. A transient ischemic attack (TIA) is a temporary interference with the blood supply to the brain lasting a few moments to several hours.
    (36:877; 17:61)

46. **(A)** The transporter should be near the patient's head so that he can converse with the patient or be available to assist the patient in an emergency such as vomiting. When the patient is on the stretcher, his feet should be pointed down hallway first.   *(5:23)*

47. **(D)** Activated glutaraldehyde penetrates into the crevices of items, is noncorrosive, does not damage lenses or cement on lensed instruments, is not absorbed by rubber and plastic, and can be reused throughout the effective activation period.   *(2:103)*

48. **(D)** A Gelpi is a self-retaining retractor.   *(6:187)*

49. **(C)** Pancreatitis is the inflammation that results when the digestive enzymes, normally secreted by the pancreas into the gastrointestinal tract, autodigest the pancreas and initiate inflammation in contiguous organs.   *(11:268)*

50. **(C)** The piston valve on the outer cannula prevents loss of carbon dioxide through the cannula after trocar removal and before scope insertion.   *(6:58)*

51. **(B)** Fistula in ano is a tiny tubular tract originating on the skin beside the anus and continuing into the anal canal.   *(7:793)*

52. **(C)** Arthrodesis is the surgical immobilization of a joint. It is often done for deformity or pain resulting from arthritis.   *(36:136; 32:522)*

53. **(A)** Solutions are steam sterilized alone and on slow exhaust. This is used so that the solutions do not boil over.   *(2:99)*

54. **(D)** A medullary canal reamer used with a Hudson brace reams the medullary canal for insertion of a Küntscher nail.   *(6:158)*

55. **(C)** Epigastric hernias are located where fatty tissue protrudes through an abdominal wall defect between the xyphoid process and the umbilicus. Surgical repair is simple and successful.   *(32:160)*

56. **(C)** In this position the entire table is tilted so that the head is higher than the feet. It is used in thyroid surgery to facilitate breathing and decrease blood supply to the operative area. It is used in gallbladder surgery to allow abdominal viscera to fall away from the epigastric area, thus giving better exposure and access.   *(2:217)*

57. **(A)** Microbial destruction is via a denaturation and coagulation of enzyme-protein in the cell.   *(32:52)*

58. **(B)** The laparoscope has a trocar which aids in its puncture through the abdominal wall.   *(32:358)*

59. **(C)** A nasogastric tube is inserted intraoperatively to maintain bowel decompression. It remains in place during the initial postoperative healing process.
    (14:75)

60. **(B)** The strength and stability of the shoulder joint are not provided by the shape of the articulating bones or its ligaments. The muscles and tendons are arranged to form a nearly complete encirclement of the joint. This arrangement is referred to as the rotator cuff and is a common site of injury to baseball pitchers.
    (38:190)

61. **(C)** For pneumonectomy, a posterolateral approach is used and the patient is placed on the table in the lateral position. A pillow is placed under the head and also between the patient's legs. The bottom leg flexed, the top straight. The bottom knee is padded. The upper arm is flexed slightly and raised above the head and supported on a raised armboard. Compression of lower arm must be avoided.   *(32:98–99, 374)*

62. **(B)** In gas sterilization, any tubing or other item with a lumen should be blown out with air to force-dry before packaging, as the water combines with the EO gas to form a harmful acid, ethylene glycol.
(2:101)

63. **(B)** The Alexander rib raspatory is double-ended. It is a periosteal on one end and a rasp on the other.
(6:236)

64. **(B)** Dissection of the gallbladder from the bed of the liver is accomplished by the use of right-angle (mixter) clamps, blunt peanut dissectors, and Metzenbaum scissors.
(32:186, 187)

65. **(B)** A self-retaining mouth gag with assorted blades is a Dingman and is frequently used in tonsillectomies and adenoidectomies.
(32:553)

66. **(C)** The storage life for muslin is 21 days or less on open shelving. It is 30 days in a closed cabinet. It is longer if it is hermetically sealed in a plastic overwrap.
(2:97)

67. **(C)** In kidney position the knee of the unaffected side is flexed to aid in stabilization and the upper leg is straight. Legs are separated with a pillow.
(2:219)

68. **(A)** The thymus gland is a bilobed organ located in the upper mediastinum posterior to the sternum and between the lungs. It plays a role in the immunity mechanism of the body.
(38:803)

69. **(A)** The islets of Langerhans manufacture insulin. They are a cluster of gland cells (endocrine) located in the pancreas. They also secrete glucagon and somatostatin.
(38:789)

70. **(A)** The sciatic nerve is the largest nerve of the body. It passes from the pelvis through the greater sciatic foramen, down the back of the thigh, where it divides into the tibial and peroneal nerves. Sciatica is severe pain in the leg along the course of the sciatic nerve felt at the back of the thigh running down the inside of the leg.
(36:1529)

71. **(B)** When in lithotomy position, legs should be raised, positioned, and lowered at the same time slowly, with no sudden movement and good support. Raising the legs simultaneously also prevents strain on the back and possible dislocation of the hips. Slow movements prevent hypotension as blood re-enters the legs.
(20:126; 11:77)

72. **(A)** A sterile pack that drops on the floor should be discarded because compression results from the fall and air and dust could enter the package. It can no longer be considered sterile.
(2:142–143)

73. **(D)** A Yankauer suction tip is used in a T&A and has a small hole at the end for directed suctioning. It is frequently used in general surgery when a limited amount of suctioning is to be done.
(17:473)

74. **(C)** Choledochotomy is done to relieve obstruction in the common bile duct. In this procedure the common bile duct is explored. If a cholangiogram is done, a radiopaque dye is inserted through a catheter to obtain x-rays.
(32:189)

75. **(C)** Great care must be taken in ligating the splenic artery and vein because they are friable. Hemorrhage is the principal hazard encountered in surgery.
(2:324)

76. **(B)** Intestinal anastomosis utilizes interrupted silk suture for the serosal muscular layer. The mucosal layer is sutured with contiuous chromic suture.
(30:408)

77. **(D)** An Esmarch bandage is applied before the pneumatic tourniquet is inflated to force blood from the extremity.
(2:371)

78. **(D)** If a solution must be poured into a sterile receptacle on a sterile field, the scrub nurse holds the receptacle away from the table or sets it near the edge of a waterproof-draped table. The circulating nurse may not pour by reaching over the sterile field. She also must be careful not to drip any solution from outside of bottle onto sterile field.
(32:48)

79. **(D)** Peroneal concerns the fibula (bone in the lower leg) and the common peroneal (lateral popliteal) nerve. Inadequately padded or improperly placed legs can cause pressure on the peroneal nerve.
(32:272; 11:77)

80. **(A)** The larynx is composed mainly of muscles and cartilages. The largest of the cartilages are the thyroid, cricoid, and epiglottic. The voice box connects the pharynx with the trachea.
(38:545, 547)

81. **(C)** The epiglottis is a leaflike structure that acts as a hinged trap door at the entrance to the larynx. It closes during swallowing to prevent aspiration of liquids or solids into the trachea.
(34:440)

82. **(B)** The paired maxillary bones unite to form the upper jawbone. The maxillae articulate with every bone of the face except the mandible (or jawbone). Each maxillary bone contains a maxillary sinus that empties into the nasal cavity.
(38:146–147)

83. **(C)** A precautionary measure in the lateral chest position is to place a sandbag under the weightbearing thorax at axillary level to relieve pressure and ensure uninhibited infusion therapy.
(2:220)

84. **(D)** A laminar flow system is a high unidirectional ventilation system which moves air either vertically or horizontally across the operative area or room, and thus controls airborne contamination.   *(2:83)*

85. **(A)** An adhesive spray or collodian is adequate over a small incision and is especially desirable under diapers, unless dressings are needed to absorb drainage.   *(2:462)*

86. **(C)** Choledochostomy is the establishment of an opening into the common bile duct by means of a drainage T tube.   *(33:208)*

87. **(D)** The direction of the cervical canal and the depth of the uterine cavity are determined by means of a graduated uterine sound.   *(32:326)*

88. **(D)** A popular method of treating patients with a peptic ulcer is by cutting the vagus nerve. The vagus nerve stimulates gastric acid, which is believed to be responsible for most peptic ulcers.   *(7:747)*

89. **(C)** Antiembolic stockings or elastic bandages may be applied to the lower extremities to prevent embolic phenomena.   *(2:66)*

90. **(A)** The OR staff should remask between patients.   *(2:123)*

91. **(B)** Benzoin may be sprayed on the skin before applying tape to increase its adhesion.   *(2:149)*

92. **(C)** A Shirodkar operation is the placement of a collar-type ligature of mersilene or Dacron at the level of the internal os to close it and prevent premature cervical dilation in a pregnancy.   *(32:328)*

93. **(B)** To produce pneumoperitoneum, a Verres needle is introduced infraumbilically into the peritoneal cavity. The gas is slowly introduced into the cavity under controlled flow and pressure.   *(2:341)*

94. **(A)** Hemostatic agents usually are packed into extremely vascular prostatic fossa to help control bleeding. Pressure from the Foley catheter balloon inserted after the closure of the urethra also helps obtain hemostasis.   *(2:360)*

95. **(C)** Electrical connection of the patient to the conductive floor is provided by a conductive strap in contact with the patient's skin, with one end of the strap fastened to the metal frame of the OR table.   *(2:287)*

96. **(B)** If CPR has been instituted and a ventricular fibrillation or tachycardia without a pulse is evident, countershock is given immediately, followed by CPR. Defibrillation affords short duration electrical shock to the heart. This stimulates the heart muscle and the heart beats.   *(2:202–204)*

97. **(C)** The humerus connects at the top with the scapula. It connects with the two forearm bones at the elbow. The two forearm bones are the ulna and the radius.   *(38:164)*

98. **(C)** Skeletal muscle tissue is attached to bones. It is striated (marked by streaks or stripes). It is voluntary meaning that movement is under conscious control.   *(38:204)*

99. **(C)** A tendon is a white fibrous cord of dense, regularly arranged connective tissue that attaches muscle to bone. When the connective tissue elements extend as a broad, flat layer, the tendon is called an aponeurosis. This structure also attaches to the coverings of bones or to another muscle.   *(38:97, 205)*

100. **(D)** Anterior-posterior repairs are more easily accomplished when done with a vaginal hysterectomy and are not contraindicated.   *(32:332)*

101. **(B)** Potentially contaminated instruments used on the cervix and vagina are placed in a discard basin and removed from the field after surgery.   *(32:335)*

102. **(A)** The pectoral girdle, or shoulder girdle, is composed of four parts: two clavicles (or collarbones) and two scapulae (or shoulder blades). The clavicle is the anterior component and articulates with the sternum at the sternoclavicular joint.   *(38:164)*

103. **(C)** The abdominal wall in the groin area is composed of two groups of muscles, fascia and muscular aponeuroses lined interiorly by peritoneum and exteriorly by skin. The superficial group (Scarpa's fascia, external and internal oblique muscles and their aponeuroses) and a deep group, (the internal oblique, transverse fascia, and peritoneum). Hernia surgery is in the groin area.   *(32:152)*

104. **(B)** The left lung is divided into a superior and inferior lobe separated by the oblique fissure. The right lung has three lobes. The oblique fissure separates the inferior lobe and the superior lobe. The horizontal fissure of the right lung subdivides the superior lobe, thus forming a middle lobe.   *(38:552)*

105. **(A)** A Hemovac is used for constant closed suction. The suction is maintained by a plastic container with a spring inside that tries to force apart the lids, thereby producing suction which is transmitted through plastic tubing. It is left in for about 3 days.   *(32:651)*

106. **(D)** In adults, the medullary cavity is the space within the diaphysis that contains the fatty yellow marrow. Yellow marrow consists primarily of fat cells and a few scattered blood cells.   *(38:125)*

107. **(D)** Syphilis is a sexually transmitted disease caused by the bacterium *Treponema pallidum*. It is acquired through sexual contact or transmitted through the placenta to the fetus. It may also be transmitted via transfusion, contact with freshly contaminated material, or by entering through a break in the skin.   *(37:723; 36:1681)*

108. **(A)** Methylene blue is used for urinary diagnostic procedures. It turns the urine a greenish blue color when used systemically. It is also used as a skin marker.   *(17:97)*

109. **(A)** Primary union (healing by first intention) occurs in clean surgical wounds aseptically made. There is a minimum of tissue destruction and tissue reaction. There are no post-op complications such as dehiscence, infection, excessive discharge, swelling, or abdominal scar formation.   *(32:125)*

110. **(B)** Normally a small amount of clear fluid is contained in the tunica vaginalis, a sac in the scrotum. When the amount increases it is known as a hydrocele. A varicocele is a congested vein; a cystocele is a herniation of the bladder through the vaginal mucosa of a female; a spermatocele is a cystic mass attached to the upper pole of the epididymis.   *(32:269)*

111. **(D)** Periosteal elevators are used to lift the periosteum from the surface of the bone. The size ranges in width and choice is dependent on the width of the surface to be removed.   *(17:308)*

112. **(B)** Cranioplasty is the repair of a skull defect resulting from trauma, malformation, or a surgical procedure.   *(32:725)*

113. **(A)** The anterior and posterior ligaments form the knee joint. The most common type of knee injury is rupture of the tibial collateral ligament, often associated with tearing of the anterior cruciate ligament and the medial meniscus (torn cartilage). It is caused by a blow to the lateral side of the knee.   *(38:194–195)*

114. **(D)** The pancreas is both an endocrine and an exocrine gland. The endocrine portion consists of cells, islets or Langerhans. It is 6 inches long with a head, tail, and a body.   *(38:421)*

115. **(C)** The physician may order it to be clamped for 4 hours and then released for 15 to 30 minutes. During the clamped time, the patient is encouraged to void.

When he can void on his own, the drainage remains clamped until it is removed.   *(7:913–914)*

116. **(B)** A calibrated ohmmeter tests conductivity of personnel and equipment.   *(2:287)*

117. **(A)** Chest drainage prevents outside air from being drawn into the pleural space during expiration. Water in the collection units seals off outside air to maintain a negative pressure within the pleural cavity. Fluids drain by gravity from the chest into the water. This system ensures complete lung expansion postoperatively.   *(2:247)*

118. **(B)** Extreme flexion of the thighs in lithotomy position impairs respiratory function by increasing intra-abdominal pressure against the diaphragm.   *(32:96)*

119. **(C)** After a vertical incision is made and extended along the medial aspect of the thigh over the femoral artery, a Weitlaner retractor is inserted into the incision.   *(32:433)*

120. **(C)** The Ellik evacuator is a double-bowl-shaped glass evacuator. It contains a trap for fragments so they cannot be washed back into the sheath of the endoscope while irrigating with pressure on the rubber-bulb attachment.   *(2:364)*

121. **(B)** Surgical interruption of selected posterior spinal roots between the ganglia and the cord is called a rhizotomy. This results in permanent loss of sensation and may be done at any spinal level. It can be performed for pain of carcinoma, tic douloureux, and other forms of tissue destruction.   *(7:1204)*

122. **(C)** Two small structures, the bulbourethral or Cowper's gland, are located below the prostate gland. They release a fluid upon sexual stimulation which lubricates the penis.   *(38:706)*

123. **(C)** Granulation tissue in third-intention healing usually forms a wide, fibrous scar. Suturing is delayed due to much tissue removal.   *(32:125–126)*

124. **(D)** *Staphylococcus aureus* is a cause of suppurative conditions, such as boils, carbuncles, and internal abscesses. It is pathogenic, gram-positive, and is transmitted due to its presence on skin and mucous membrane.   *(36:1618)*

125. **(B)** Mannitol is a most effective osmotic diuretic and valuable in reducing intercranial pressure or edema. It may be given prophylactically to prevent renal failure. It also reduces intraocular pressure.   *(2:144)*

126. **(B)** The clavicles or collarbones are the long slender bones with a double curvature. The medial end of the clavicle articulates with the sternum. The lateral end articulates with the scapula. *(38:164)*

127. **(A)** Cortisone is used as an anti-inflammatory. It is a hormone isolated from the cortex of the adrenal gland and it is prepared synthetically. *(36:389)*

128. **(B)** The clinical manifestations of hemorrhage are pulse increase, fall in temperature, respirations rapid and deep, and fall in blood pressure. The patient is apprehensive and restless. He or she may be thirsty. The skin is cold, moist, and pale. *(7:370)*

129. **(C)** All flammable gases and vapors except ethylene are heavier than air and settle to the floor when released. Electrical fixtures and outlets located less than 5 feet above the ground must meet rigid explosion code requirements. *(2:116)*

130. **(B)** Carpel tunnel syndrome is a disease of the hand resulting in compression of the median nerve within the carpal tunnel. The necessary surgery is release of the bound down nerve and relief of pressure. *(17:321)*

131. **(C)** Chronic irritation can result in an abnormal whitening of the mucous membrane of the lip or tongue. This condition, known as leukoplakia, is thought to be a precancerous lesion and is seen most frequently in heavy smokers. *(2:421)*

132. **(C)** Phimosis is a condition in which the foreskin is narrowed so that it cannot be retracted over the glans (head of the penis). *(7:1029)*

133. **(B)** Second-degree burns include all epidermis and varying degrees or depths of corium. It is characterized by blister, pain, and redness. Hair follicles and sebaceous glands may be destroyed. *(2:453)*

134. **(D)** Anaerobes are those microbes that prefer to live without oxygen. Facultative anaerobes can survive in the presence of oxygen. Obligate anaerobes die immediately. *(8:61)*

135. **(A)** The testes produce sperm and secrete the male sex hormone, testosterone. The vas deferens stores sperm up to several weeks. *(34:615–616)*

136. **(A)** The inner tunic of the eye consists of the retina, which contains the receptor cells of sight. Its function is image formation. It covers the choroid. *(38:382)*

137. **(C)** Idiopathic diseases—the term idiopathic means undetermined cause. Of the many examples of idiopathic disease, hypertension is perhaps the most common. For 90% of persons with hypertension, there is no known cause. *(37:350)*

138. **(B)** Drugs that exert a selective action on the smooth muscled uterus to promote contractions are called oxytocics. They exert a stronger effect on the fundus than they do on the cervix. *(36:1200)*

139. **(C)** After an opening is made into the anterior bladder and the opening is extended with scissors, a Mason-Judd self-retaining bladder retractor is inserted and the bladder is explored. *(32:276)*

140. **(D)** During a lumbar laminectomy, one or two Beckman-Adson self-retaining retractors are used to expose the bone structure of the spinal column. *(32:764)*

141. **(C)** Adhesions are a common development after repeated attacks of PID and eventually may necessitate removal of uterus, tubes, and ovaries. *(7:999)*

142. **(D)** A Hakim valve system is used to direct the flow of cerebrospinal fluid and regulate ventricular fluid pressure by opening within a preset range and draining excess fluid into the atrium or the peritoneum. *(32:761)*

143. **(C)** Spinal fusion may be effected by use of an autogenous graft from the crest of the patient's ilium. Cancellous bone is preferred to cortical bone. *(2:376)*

144. **(B)** Hallux valgus, a lateral deviation in the position of the great toe, increases the prominence of the adjoining metatarsal head. Pressure at the metatarsophalangeal joint causes inflammation, which creates formation of an exostosis (bunion) beneath the bursa and joint capsule. *(2:375)*

145. **(C)** The anterior one-sixth of the outer tunic bulges forward and is known as the transparent cornea, which helps focus light rays and serves as the window of the eye. *(21:414)*

146. **(D)** Stimulation of the adrenal gland produces hormones including epinephrine which prepare the body to meet emergency situations. Synthetic "adrenaline" is used to check hemorrhage and to relieve asthmatic attacks. *(36:563)*

147. **(A)** Nosocomial infections are hospital-acquired infections. Infection which the patient did not have prior to admission in the hospital. *(32:39)*

148. **(B)** Cardiac compression is effected by placement of heel of one hand over the lower third of the sternum, above xiphoid process (1 to 1.5 inches). The other hand is on top of it. Fingers are arched upward so as not to exert force on the ribs. *(2:206)*

149. **(C)** The edges of anything that encloses sterile contents are considered unsterile. *(2:88)*

150. **(C)** The Gibbons silicone indwelling stent catheter is inserted for long-term drainage in a wide variety of benign and malignant diseases causing ureteral obstruction. *(2:355)*

151. **(C)** Colpocleisis obliterates the vagina by denuding and approximating the anterior and posterior walls. Colpocleisis (Le Fort) is reserved for elderly patients or poor-risk patients. *(2:344)*

152. **(C)** Trigeminal neuralgia (tic douloureux) is a neuralgia affecting the third, fourth, and fifth cranial nerves. It causes excruciating and piercing pain. *(32:710)*

153. **(D)** A Harrington retractor is used in deep abdominal surgery. All of the others can be found in a dilation and curettage. *(32:313)*

154. **(A)** Anterior colporrhaphy is performed to correct prolapse of the anterior vaginal vault and repair herniation of the bladder into the vaginal canal. *(2:343)*

155. **(C)** The frontal sinus is approached by making an incision above the eyebrow on the affected side. Diseased tissue is then removed, the sinus cavity is cleansed, and drainage is instituted. *(32:626)*

156. **(C)** An incision is made under the upper lip in a Caldwell-Luc procedure. An opening is created into the maxillary sinus, after which the infected contents of the sinus are removed. To promote good drainage a large nasoantral window is created. *(32:288)*

157. **(C)** A Küntscher or Schneider nail can be used to immobilize a fracture of the femoral shaft. *(32:505)*

158. **(D)** The vagus nerve, X, is the longest cranial nerve. It supplies most of the organs in the thoracic and abdominal cavities. This nerve also contains secretory fibers to glands that produce digestive juices and other secretions. *(38:336)*

159. **(A)** The under-the-tongue normal body temperature is 98.6°F. This is 37°C. Rectal temperature degree reading is likely to be 0.5 to 1.0° above the oral. *(36:1702)*

160. **(B)** After the skin incision, place the knife in a specimen basin. The inside of this basin is considered contaminated so the scrub should refrain from touching anything else that is put in it. *(2:140)*

161. **(D)** The Levin tube is a common rubber or plastic nasogastric tube. It is inserted through the nostril down into the stomach or small intestine to remove flatus, fluids, or other contents. *(2:246)*

162. **(B)** A dislocation is a complete displacement of one articular surface of a joint from another. A subluxation is a partial dislocation. *(32:464)*

163. **(B)** Continuous irrigation of the bladder is necessary during cystoscopy to distend the walls for visualization and to wash out blood, tissue, and stone fragments. *(2:363)*

164. **(C)** Debridement, the excision of necrotic tissue, is accomplished with a scalpel, an electrosurgical knife, a dermatome, or a laser beam. After a good vascular supply is located, a full-thickness or split-thickness graft can be used to preserve and cover the area. *(2:454)*

165. **(D)** The aging process causes a sagging or relaxation of eyelid skin and the orbital septum. As the latter becomes weaker, it allows periorbital fat to bulge. These changes are perceived as baggy eyelids. The surgical repair of this condition is blepharoplasty. *(32:569)*

166. **(C)** A pterygium is a fleshy, triangular encroachment onto the cornea. It occurs nasally and tends to be bilateral. If it encroaches on the visual axis it is removed surgically. *(32:698)*

167. **(A)** The hypothalamus contains neurosecretions that are of importance in the control of certain metabolic activities. These include maintenance of water balance, sugar and fat metabolism, regulation of body temperature, and secretion of releasing and inhibiting hormones. *(36:813; 27:85)*

168. **(D)** The ulna is the medial bone of the forearm (little finger side). On the proximal end of the ulna is the olecranon, a large process of the ulna projecting behind the elbow joint. It forms the bony prominence of the elbow. *(36:1156)*

169. **(A)** The ovarian follicle is the ova and their surrounding tissue in various stages of development. The ovaries produce ova, discharge ova (ovulation), and secrete the female hormones (progesterone, estrogens, and relaxin). *(38:709)*

170. **(C)** The paired broad ligaments are double folds of parietal peritoneum attaching the uterus to either side of the pelvic cavity. The uterosacrals connect the uterus to the sacrum. The cardinals maintain the position of the uterus and keep it from dropping into the vagina. The round ligaments are bands of fibrous connective tissue which extend from just below the uterine tubes to a portion of the external genitalia. *(38:713)*

171. **(A)** Carbohydrates are a basic source of energy. They are also known as sugars and starches. The principle function is to provide the most readily available source of energy to sustain life.   *(36:264; 38:42)*

172. **(D)** Bradycardia is slowness of the heartbeat, less than 60 beats per minute. Sinus bradycardia is seen normally in athletes or secondary to certain drugs (digitalis or morphine).   *(2:162; 7:527)*

173. **(D)** If a glove is pricked by a needle or snagged by an instrument, the glove should be changed at once and the needle or instrument discarded.   *(2:141)*

174. **(C)** The CO_2 laser operates in the middle of the infrared portion of the spectrum and is delivered to the tissue coupled to the operating microscope or with the aid of articulating mirrors and hand probes. CO_2 laser emissions are heavily absorbed by water.   *(28:390)*

175. **(C)** Progesterone is a hormone secreted by the corpus luteum. It is essential in the implantation of the fertilized ovum.   *(32:308)*

176. **(C)** Iridencleisis is an opening created between the anterior chamber and the space beneath the conjunctiva, thereby bypassing the trabecular meshwork and relieving intraocular pressure.   *(33:116)*

177. **(C)** Through microscopic visualization, the aural speculum is inserted in the canal. Using a sharp myringotomy knife, a small curved incision is made in the posterioinferior quadrant or the pars tina, and the thickened membrane is cut.   *(32:604)*

178. **(B)** A perfusionist aids in temperature, arterial and venous pressure, and blood gas monitoring, as well as peripheral tissue perfusion (passing of fluid) monitoring during a cardiopulmonary bypass.   *(7:553)*

179. **(D)** The closed glove method is preferred because it affords assurance against contamination. This technique cannot be safely used for glove change during an operation.   *(2:128, 133)*

180. **(D)** Accelerated respirations occur in febrile diseases. They decrease in diabetic coma, conditions that cause intracranial pressure, shock, poisoning, etc.   *(36:1476–1477)*

181. **(B)** In second intention, the wound is left open and heals from the bottom up. Scar formation is excessive. Infection, trauma, loss of tissue, or poor approximation of tissue is present.   *(2:240)*

182. **(A)** The middle ear consists of an air-filled space in the temporal bone called the tympanic cavity. This separates the external and inner ears. Three small bones or auditory ossicles – the malleus (hammer), incus (anvil), and the stapes (stirrup) – are attached to the wall of the tympanic cavity by tiny ligaments.   *(38:389)*

183. **(B)** The temperature taken rectally is usually from 0.5 to 1.0°F higher than by mouth, and the axillary temperature is about 0.5°F lower than by the mouth. Body temperature is a result of the balance between heat production and heat loss.   *(36:1702)*

184. **(A)** The right glove is usually done first. Hold the palm of the glove toward the person, stretching the cuff and holding your thumbs out so as to avoid touching the hand. Unfold the everted cuff over the cuff of the sleeve.   *(2:132)*

185. **(B)** Tinnitus is a very common condition of the ear. It can be unilateral or bilateral. Many pathologic conditions can produce tinnitus, from a plug of ear wax to otosclerosis.   *(33:440)*

186. **(C)** Laser is an acronym for light amplification by stimulated emission of radiation. It is a device that produces an intense, coherent directional beam of light by stimulated electronic or molecular transition to a lower energy level.   *(28:390)*

187. **(B)** When a patient has a breast biopsy and immediate extended operation, two separate prepping, draping, and instrument sets are necessary.   *(2:317–318)*

188. **(B)** Blood pressure sounds are heard over the brachial artery. The bell of the stethoscope is placed over the brachial artery below the blood pressure cuff. The first sound heard is the systolic pressure. The sound at which the sound is no longer heard is the diastolic.   *(36:213–214)*

189. **(D)** Leukocytes (white blood cells) are phagocytic which is a response to tissue destruction by bacteria. They ingest bacteria and dispose of dead matter. They release the enzyme lysozyme which destroys certain bacteria.   *(38:440)*

190. **(B)** Ductless glands, endocrine glands, secrete hormones internally discharged into blood or lymph and is circulated to all parts of the body. Hormones, the active principles of the glands produces effects on tissues (pituitary, thyroid, and parathyroid, adrenals, islets of Langerhans, and the gonads).   *(36:542)*

191. **(B)** The left atrium is the receiving chamber for blood from the lungs. The blood is carried to the left atrium by four pulmonary veins.   *(36:152)*

192. **(B)** The liver's main function is the production of bile, a thick, yellow-green fluid. Bile is particularly an excretory product and partially a digestive secretion.   *(38:607)*

193. **(C)** The carpal tunnel is located along the volar surface of the wrist. The median nerve, superficial and deep finger flexors, and the long thumb flexor tendon all pass through the carpal tunnel before entering the hand. *(32:583–584)*

194. **(C)** Cytologic specimen collectors, such as Clerf or Lukens traps, are used to hold endoscopic secretions as they are obtained. *(32:365)*

195. **(C)** With vascular forceps and a #11 blade, an arteriotomy is effected and extended with a Potts-Smith vascular scissor. *(32:434)*

196. **(C)** Evisceration is a protrusion of viscera through abdominal incision. During surgery meticulous attention to sterile technique, hemostasis, tissue handling, and approximation and selection of wound closure materials are all precautions which could prevent this from occurring. It is generally attributed to a poor healing process induced by poor nutrition, poor circulation, and the improper formation of thrombin. *(2:499–500)*

197. **(C)** The first 10 or 12 inches of the small intestine is called the duodenum. It joins with the jejunum which is 8 feet long. The jejunum joins with the ileum which is 12 feet long. *(38:610)*

198. **(D)** *Escherichia coli* live in the colon or large intestine. A colostomy is an opening of some portion of the colon on the abdominal surface. An adjacent wound could be contaminated with *E. coli*. *(37:12)*

199. **(D)** A liter is a metric fluid measurement equivalent to 1000 milliliters or approximately 1000 cubic centimeters. This is 1.0567 quart. Volume should be expressed in ml rather than cc. *(36:967)*

200. **(A)** Urinary catheterization requires aseptic technique. The integrity of the balloon is checked by inflating it with the correct amount of sterile water or air prior to insertion. After insertion, the bladder is drained and the balloon is then inflated. *(2:221–222)*

201. **(D)** Proper setting for an adult leg is 400 to 500 mm Hg. Accurate tourniquet time must be recorded and periodically announced to the surgeon. *(32:461)*

202. **(B)** Crushing a urinary calculus with a lithotrite is referred to as litholapaxy. A lithotrite is introduced through the urethra, and the stone is crushed and removed. A cystoscope is introduced into the urethra for introduction of the lithotrite. *(2:356)*

203. **(C)** A vasectomy is the ligation and transection of a section of the vas deferens. It is performed if a patient has recurrent acute epididymitis. Epididymectomy is performed only if the recurrent attacks are incapacitating and chronic. *(7:1031)*

204. **(B)** The umbilicus is considered contaminated. Either come back to the umbilicus and scrub it before discarding the prep sponge or use a separate sponge on the umbilicus only. It should be cleansed thoroughly with cotton applicators. *(2:224)*

205. **(C)** Below the fundus of the stomach the region narrows as it approaches the junction to the small intestine. This is the pylorus or distal portion of the stomach. *(38:597)*

206. **(B)** Lasix (furosemide) is a diuretic. A diuretic increases the secretion of urine. *(32:243)*

207. **(C)** The average capacity of the bladder is 700 to 800 ml. When the amount of urine in the bladder exceeds 200 to 400 ml, the impulses are transmitted which initiate a conscious desire to expel urine. Although emptying of the bladder is controlled by reflex, it may be initiated voluntarily and stopped at will. *(38:678)*

208. **(C)** The anus is considered a contaminated (dirty) area. The prep is done of the surrounding area first. The anus itself is last. *(17:82)*

209. **(A)** When changing a gown during an operation, the gown is always removed first with the circulator pulling the gown off inside-out. The gloves are removed using glove-to-glove then skin-to-skin technique. A rescrub is not necessary. *(2:132–133)*

210. **(C)** Skin meshers cut small slits in the graft. When expanded, the slits become diamond-shaped openings. This permits expansion of the graft to cover three times as large an area as the original graft obtained from the donor site. *(2:447)*

211. **(A)** Ninety percent of calculi in the urinary tract are calcium-formed; uric acid forms 8% and cystine causes 1 to 3%. Small amounts of mixed stones are found. *(7:941)*

212. **(A)** Inside the kidney, the ureter expands to form a basin which receives urine collected by the collecting tubules in the medulla. This space is called the renal pelvis or basin. It is a cavity in the center of the kidney and the calyces open into it. *(38:799)*

213. **(C)** The kidneys are held in position by connective tissue (renal fascia) and masses of adipose tissue (renal fat) which surrounds them. Inadequate renal fascia may cause ptosis or floating kidney. *(38:358)*

214. **(A)** A culture identifies the suspected organism causing infection. Sensitivity determines the susceptibility of the patient's bacterial infection to antibiotics or antibacterials. The specimen obtained from the patient is cultured in various liquid dilutions of the drugs or on solid media containing various concentrations of the drug on disks placed on surface of the media. The disk-type is not completely reliable.   *(36:405, 1545)*

215. **(A)** The most frequently used scrub agent is povidone-iodine (an iodophor).   *(2:109, 126)*

216. **(C)** A Joseph's saw is bayonet-like in design and is used for nasal procedures. The Alexander, Langenbeck, and Lebsche are used for chest procedures.   *(32:359–360)*

217. **(B)** Delayed union signifies that a specific fracture has not healed in the time considered average for that fracture. Delayed union must not be considered non-union until the healing process has ceased without bony union.   *(32:467)*

218. **(A)** A guide wire or pin is placed in the neck and head of the proximal fragment of the fracture. This determines the final position of the implant to be used.   *(32:493)*

219. **(D)** The primary source of estrogen is the ovaries. Estrogen is responsible for the development of female secondary sex characteristics. Progesterone is also produced in the ovaries.   *(38:424)*

220. **(A)** The infundibulum is the funnel-shaped open end of each tube from which the fimbriae extend. It lies close to the ovary but not attached to it. It is surrounded by fimbriae.   *(38:70)*

221. **(B)** A stoma may be sealed from the operative site with a self-adhering towel. If this is not done, come back to the stoma area last or use a separate sponge on the area. This helps to prevent contamination of incision site.   *(2:224)*

222. **(B)** Antiembolic stockings or an elastic bandage may be ordered applied to lower extremities prior to surgery to prevent thrombus formation. This is often done prior to abdominal or pelvic procedures, and for patients who have varicosities, who are prone to thrombus formation, or who have a history of embolus, and some geriatric patients.   *(2:66)*

223. **(B)** Skin cannot be sterilized but it can be rendered surgically clean (the number of bacteria is greatly reduced) by the scrub procedure.   *(4:58)*

224. **(D)** In laparoscopy, carbon dioxide is introduced via a Verres needle to create a pneumoperitoneum.   *(32:334)*

225. **(C)** Skeletal traction, applied by Crutchfield tongs inserted in the parietal eminence of the skull, is generally used for reduction of fractures and dislocations of the cervical vertebrae.   *(24:198)*

226. **(B)** Hepatitis is an inflammation of the liver. Hepatitis A, infectious hepatitis, is spread by the oral-intestinal route and is caused by hepatitis A virus. Common modes are contaminated food and water and shellfish from contaminated water. Hepatitis B, serum hepatitis is associated with the blood. Common transmission modes are blood transfusions and contaminated equipment such as syringes.   *(37:562–623)*

227. **(B)** *Staphylococcus* is transmitted by the skin and mucous membrane. It is especially common to the nose and mouth.   *(36:1618; 32:41)*

228. **(D)** Spores remain dormant while the conditions for its growth are unfavorable. Its thick coating protects it from temperature extremes or strong chemicals.   *(17:22)*

229. **(C)** Catheters are available in 5 or 30 cc balloons. A third lumen can be used for irrigation. Following some types of GU surgery, it is important to irrigate any clots or debris from the bladder.   *(2:375)*

230. **(B)** If a towel clip must be removed, discard it from the sterile setup without touching the points, as they are considered contaminated. The area from which it was removed is covered with another sterile drape.   *(2:232)*

231. **(A)** The Hohmann retractor's shape makes it an invaluable tool for maintaining subluxation of the femoral head in a total hip replacement.   *(32:500)*

232. **(A)** *Pseudomonas* infection occurs in postburn patients. They are opportunists and the burn patients are susceptible because their skin is no longer an effective barrier to microorganisms.   *(37:507, 515)*

233. **(B)** Breast biopsy usually requires frozen section which is not placed in formalin. Kidney stones are sent dry so the chemical composition is not altered. Bronchial washings are sent down in the specimen collection unit as soon as possible and formalin is not used on them. Tonsils would be sent in formalin.   *(17:198, 347)*

234. **(A)** A tort is a legal wrong committed by one person involving injury to another person or loss of or damage to personal property. When a tort has been committed, a patient or family member may institute a civil action against the person or persons who caused the injury, loss, or damage.   *(2:503)*

235. **(D)** Harrington rods are implanted into the spine by clips that hold onto the laminae. They are used in combination with (rather than as a replacement for) the external methods of scoliosis support.   *(24:376)*

236. **(C)** Pentothal sodium is a barbiturate. It is a short-acting drug used for induction prior to administration of more potent anesthetics such as inhalants. It can also be used for short procedures not requiring relaxation.   *(2:172)*

237. **(D)** When a heated blanket is used, a sheet should be placed between the patient and the blanket. The blanket temperature should not exceed 42°C (107.6°F).   *(19:311)*

238. **(D)** Legally, the patient's condition is confidential information. The case should not be discussed outside of the OR. The patient's right to privacy exists either by statutory or common law.   *(2:505)*

239. **(A)** Protect the gloved hands by cuffing the end of the sheet over them.   *(2:231)*

240. **(B)** Located in the tarsal plate of the eyelid, the Meibomian gland may inflame and require surgical removal. It is known as a chalazion.   *(32:666)*

241. **(D)** Secobarbital is a barbiturate given preoperatively for its hypnotic effect to induce sleep. It also acts as a sedative. This assures that the patient gets a good night's sleep before surgery.   *(17:68)*

242. **(D)** Bowel technique is utilized when a contaminated area of the intestinal tract is entered, and may be discontinued when the bowel has been anastomosed.   *(11:210)*

243. **(C)** Dupuytren's contracture is a progressive contracture of the palmar fascia. It causes flexion of the little finger, the ring finger, and frequently the middle fingers, rendering them useless.   *(7:1339)*

244. **(A)** Disposable suction tubing is recommended. However, if tubing is reused special care must be given to cleaning the lumen prior to placing tubing with instruments for terminal sterilization. Suction a detergent-disinfectant solution through the lumen.   *(2:155)*

245. **(C)** Each needle is accounted for as the surgeon finishes with it and its integrity is checked. The surgeon is told immediately if a needle is broken so that both pieces can be retrieved. In the event that the pieces are not found, an x-ray is taken to locate the missing portions.   *(2:140)*

246. **(B)** Heparin is an anticoagulant. It acts to inhibit the reaction wherein prothrombin is converted to thrombin. The dosage is adjusted to minimize the tendency of blood to clot in vessels.   *(2:243)*

247. **(D)** Neo-Synephrine (phenylephrine HCl) is a mydriatic. It dilates the pupil thereby facilitating examination of the retina and also lens removal.   *(17:435)*

248. **(D)** The phrase means "the thing speaks for itself" and is frequently applied to injuries sustained by patient while in the OR. Three conditions must exist: (1) The type of injury does not ordinarily occur without a negligent act. (2) The injury was caused by the conduct within the control of the person or persons being sued. (3) The injured person could not have contributed to the negligence or voluntarily assumed the risk.   *(2:504)*

249. **(C)** The sterile team members discard gown, gloves, caps, masks, and shoe covers because these items should remain in the contaminated area.   *(2:156)*

250. **(B)** Pilocarpine is used to constrict the pupil to reduce intraocular pressure. In cataract surgery it is used to help prevent the loss of vitreous.   *(17:435)*

PRACTICE TEST SUBJECT LIST

BASIC SCIENCES

A. Terminology: 5, 10, 18, 23, 28, 33, 38, 45, 52, 60

B. Anatomy and Physiology: 68, 69, 70, 80, 81, 82, 97, 98, 99, 102, 103, 104, 106, 113, 114, 122, 126, 135, 136, 145, 146, 158, 167, 168, 169, 170, 171, 182, 189, 190, 191, 192, 197, 205, 207, 212, 213, 219, 220

C. Microbiology: 107, 124, 127, 134, 137, 147, 198, 226, 227, 228, 232

D. Pharmacology: 108, 125, 199, 206, 236, 237, 240, 246, 247, 250

E. Wound Healing: 109, 123, 133, 181, 196

PATIENT CARE

A. Pre-Op Routine: 4, 11, 17, 19

B. Transportation: 24, 29, 34, 44, 46

C. Positioning: 56, 61, 67, 71, 79, 83

D. Related Nursing Procedures: 96, 115, 128, 148, 159, 172, 180, 183, 188, 200, 204, 208, 214, 221, 222, 229, 233

E. Medical/Legal: 9, 234, 238, 245, 248

ASEPTIC TECHNIQUE AND ENVIRONMENTAL CONTROL

A. Sterilization, Disinfection, and Antisepsis: 3, 12, 16, 20, 25, 30, 35, 40, 43, 47, 53, 57

B. Packaging and Dispensing of Supplies: 62, 66, 72, 78

C. Environmental Control: 8, 84, 90, 95, 116, 129

D. Aseptic Technique in General Procedures: 149, 160, 173, 179, 184, 187, 209, 215, 223, 230, 239, 242, 244, 249

SUPPLIES AND EQUIPMENT

A. Sutures and Needles—Classification: 2, 13, 15, 21, 26, 31

B. Instruments—Classification: 7, 36, 42, 48, 50, 54, 58, 63, 65, 73

C. Dressing and Packings: 77, 85, 89, 91

D. Catheters, Drains, Tubes, and Collecting Mechanisms: 94, 105, 117, 150, 161

E. Equipment: 174, 178, 186, 201, 210, 224

SURGICAL PROCEDURES

A. General Surgery: 1, 6, 14, 22, 27, 32, 37, 39, 41, 49, 51, 55, 59, 64, 74, 75, 76, 86, 88

B. Gynecologic Procedures: 87, 92, 93, 100, 101, 118, 138, 141, 151, 153, 154, 175

C. Eye, Ear, Nose, Throat, and Plastic Surgery: 131, 155, 156, 164, 165, 166, 176, 177, 185, 241

D. Genitourinary Procedures: 110, 120, 132, 139, 163, 202, 203, 211

E. Thoracic, Cardiovascular, and Peripheral Vascular Procedures: 119, 194, 195, 216

F. Orthopedics, Plaster: 111, 143, 144, 157, 162, 193, 217, 218, 225, 231, 235, 243

G. Neurosurgery: 112, 121, 130, 140, 142, 152

References

1. American Heart Association: Student Manual for Basic Life Support. Dallas, Texas, 1981.
2. Atkinson L J, Kohn M: Berry and Kohn's Introduction to Operating Room Technique, 5th ed. New York, McGraw-Hill, 1978.
3. Austrin M: Learn Medical Technicology, Step by Step, 5th ed. St. Louis, C. V. Mosby, 1983.
4. Bergersen B: Pharmacology in Nursing, 15th ed. St. Louis, C. V. Mosby, 1982.
5. Brooks S: Fundamentals of Operating Room Nursing, 2nd ed. St. Louis, C. V. Mosby, 1979.
6. Brooks S: Instrumentation for the Operating Room – A Photographic Manual, 2nd ed. St. Louis, C. V. Mosby, 1983.
7. Brunner L, Suddarth D: Textbook of Medical Surgical Nursing, 5th ed. Philadelphia, Lippincott, 1984.
8. Burton G: Microbiology for the Health Sciences. Philadelphia, Lippincott, 1983.
9. Chabner D-E: The Language of Medicine. Philadelphia, Saunders, 1985.
10. Cooley D, Wukasch D: Techniques in Vascular Surgery. Philadelphia, Saunders, 1979.
11. Crooks L O: Operating Room Techniques for the Surgical Team. Boston, Little, Brown, 1979.
12. Debakey M, Goitok A: The Living Heart. New York, David McKay, 1979.
13. Dubay E, Grubb R: Infection Prevention and Control, 2nd ed. St. Louis, C. V. Mosby, 1978.
14. Ethicon Manual: Nursing Care of the Patient in the O.R., 1975.
15. Ethicon Manual: Suture Use Manual: Use and Handling of Sutures and Needles, 1977.
16. Ethicon Manual: The Human Body: Its Major Systems and Their Function, 1975.
17. Fuller J: Surgical Technology – Principles and Practices. Philadelphia, Saunders, 1981.
18. Green L, Segura J: Transurethral Surgery. Philadelphia, Saunders, 1979.
19. Groah L K: Operating Room Nursing – The Perioperative Role. Reston Publishing, 1983.
20. Gruendemann B, Casterton S, Hesterly S et al: The Surgical Patient – Behavioral Concepts for the Operating Room Nurse, 2nd ed. St. Louis, C. V. Mosby, 1977.
21. Hole J H Jr: Human Anatomy and Physiology, 2nd ed. Dubuque, Iowa, William C. Brown, 1984.
22. Jorow M: The Central Service Technician at Work. New York, Springer-Verlag, 1975.
23. Lach J: O.R. Nursing: Preoperative Care and Draping Technique. Chicago, Kendall, 1974.
24. Larson C, Gould M: Orthopedic Nursing, 9th ed. St. Louis, C. V. Mosby, 1978.
25. LeMaitre G, Finnegan J: The Patient in Surgery – A Guide for Nurses, 4th ed. Philadelphia, Saunders, 1980.
26. Mayor G, Zingg E: Urologic Surgery. New York, Wiley, 1976.
27. Memmler R, Wood D: Structure and Function of the Human Body, 3rd ed. Philadelphia, Lippincott, 1983.
28. Mid-America Vocational Curriculum Consortium: Surgical Technology Series – Surgical Procedures. Stillwater, Okla, 1985.
29. Montgomery W: Surgery of the Upper Respiratory System, Vol. 1, 2nd ed. Philadelphia, Lea & Febiger, 1979.
30. Nora P F: Operative Surgery Principles and Techniques. Philadelphia, Lea & Febiger, 1980.
31. Rexilois B: Chest Drainage and Suction. Philadelphia, F. A. Davis, 1977.
32. Rhodes G, Ballinger: Alexander's Care of the Patient in Surgery, 7th ed. St. Louis, C. V. Mosby, 1983.
33. Saunders, Havener, Keith, Havener: Nursing Care in Eye, Ear, Nose and Throat Disorders, 4th ed. St. Louis, C. V. Mosby, 1979.
34. Silverstein A: Human Anatomy and Physiology, 2nd ed. New York, Wiley, 1983.
35. Stroumtsos O: Perspectives on Suture. New York, Davis and Geck, 1978.

36. Taber's Cyclopedic Medical Dictionary, 15th ed. Philadelphia, F. A. Davis, 1985.

37. Tortora G, Furke B, Case C: Microbiology, An Introduction. Menlo Park, Calif, Benjamin Cummings, 1982.

38. Tortora G, Anagnostakos N: Principles of Anatomy and Physiology, 4th ed. New York, Harper & Row, 1984.

39. Wilson M, Mizer H, Morello J: Microbiology in Patient Care, 3rd ed. New York, Macmillan, 1979.

NAME _____
Last   First   Middle

ADDRESS _____
Street

City   State   Zip

DIRECTIONS Mark your social security number from top to bottom in the appropriate boxes on the right. Refer to the introduction to the book for more information.

MAKE ERASURES COMPLETE

PLEASE USE NO.2 PENCIL ONLY.

PAGE 1 2
TYPE 1 2 3 4 5

1 A B C D E 2 A B C D E 3 A B C D E 4 A B C D E 5 A B C D E 6 A B C D E 7 A B C D E 8 A B C D E

9 A B C D E 10 A B C D E 11 A B C D E 12 A B C D E 13 A B C D E 14 A B C D E 15 A B C D E 16 A B C D E

17 A B C D E 18 A B C D E 19 A B C D E 20 A B C D E 21 A B C D E 22 A B C D E 23 A B C D E 24 A B C D E

25 A B C D E 26 A B C D E 27 A B C D E 28 A B C D E 29 A B C D E 30 A B C D E 31 A B C D E 32 A B C D E

33 A B C D E 34 A B C D E 35 A B C D E 36 A B C D E 37 A B C D E 38 A B C D E 39 A B C D E 40 A B C D E

41 A B C D E 42 A B C D E 43 A B C D E 44 A B C D E 45 A B C D E 46 A B C D E 47 A B C D E 48 A B C D E

49 A B C D E 50 A B C D E 51 A B C D E 52 A B C D E 53 A B C D E 54 A B C D E 55 A B C D E 56 A B C D E

57 A B C D E 58 A B C D E 59 A B C D E 60 A B C D E 61 A B C D E 62 A B C D E 63 A B C D E 64 A B C D E

65 A B C D E 66 A B C D E 67 A B C D E 68 A B C D E 69 A B C D E 70 A B C D E 71 A B C D E 72 A B C D E

73 A B C D E 74 A B C D E 75 A B C D E 76 A B C D E 77 A B C D E 78 A B C D E 79 A B C D E 80 A B C D E

81 A B C D E 82 A B C D E 83 A B C D E 84 A B C D E 85 A B C D E 86 A B C D E 87 A B C D E 88 A B C D E

89 A B C D E 90 A B C D E 91 A B C D E 92 A B C D E 93 A B C D E 94 A B C D E 95 A B C D E 96 A B C D E

97 A B C D E 98 A B C D E 99 A B C D E 100 A B C D E 101 A B C D E 102 A B C D E 103 A B C D E 104 A B C D E

105 A B C D E 106 A B C D E 107 A B C D E 108 A B C D E 109 A B C D E 110 A B C D E 111 A B C D E 112 A B C D E

113 A B C D E 114 A B C D E 115 A B C D E 116 A B C D E 117 A B C D E 118 A B C D E 119 A B C D E 120 A B C D E

121 A B C D E 122 A B C D E 123 A B C D E 124 A B C D E 125 A B C D E 126 A B C D E 127 A B C D E 128 A B C D E

129 A B C D E 130 A B C D E 131 A B C D E 132 A B C D E 133 A B C D E 134 A B C D E 135 A B C D E 136 A B C D E

137 A B C D E 138 A B C D E 139 A B C D E 140 A B C D E 141 A B C D E 142 A B C D E 143 A B C D E 144 A B C D E

145 A B C D E 146 A B C D E 147 A B C D E 148 A B C D E 149 A B C D E 150 A B C D E 151 A B C D E 152 A B C D E

153 A B C D E 154 A B C D E 155 A B C D E 156 A B C D E 157 A B C D E 158 A B C D E 159 A B C D E 160 A B C D E

SOC SEC NUMBER

		0	1	2	3	4	5	6	7	8	9
S	N	0	1	2	3	4	5	6	7	8	9
O	U	0	1	2	3	4	5	6	7	8	9
C	M	0	1	2	3	4	5	6	7	8	9
	B	0	1	2	3	4	5	6	7	8	9
S	E	0	1	2	3	4	5	6	7	8	9
E	R	0	1	2	3	4	5	6	7	8	9
C		0	1	2	3	4	5	6	7	8	9
		0	1	2	3	4	5	6	7	8	9
		0	1	2	3	4	5	6	7	8	9

PAGE 1 2
TYPE 1 2 3 4 5

161 A B C D E 162 A B C D E 163 A B C D E 164 A B C D E 165 A B C D E 166 A B C D E 167 A B C D E 168 A B C D E

169 A B C D E 170 A B C D E 171 A B C D E 172 A B C D E 173 A B C D E 174 A B C D E 175 A B C D E 176 A B C D E

177 A B C D E 178 A B C D E 179 A B C D E 180 A B C D E 181 A B C D E 182 A B C D E 183 A B C D E 184 A B C D E

185 A B C D E 186 A B C D E 187 A B C D E 188 A B C D E 189 A B C D E 190 A B C D E 191 A B C D E 192 A B C D E

93 A B C D E 194 A B C D E 195 A B C D E 196 A B C D E 197 A B C D E 198 A B C D E 199 A B C D E 200 A B C D E

201 A B C D E 202 A B C D E 203 A B C D E 204 A B C D E 205 A B C D E 206 A B C D E 207 A B C D E 208 A B C D E

209 A B C D E 210 A B C D E 211 A B C D E 212 A B C D E 213 A B C D E 214 A B C D E 215 A B C D E 216 A B C D E

217 A B C D E 218 A B C D E 219 A B C D E 220 A B C D E 221 A B C D E 222 A B C D E 223 A B C D E 224 A B C D E

225 A B C D E 226 A B C D E 227 A B C D E 228 A B C D E 229 A B C D E 230 A B C D E 231 A B C D E 232 A B C D E

233 A B C D E 234 A B C D E 235 A B C D E 236 A B C D E 237 A B C D E 238 A B C D E 239 A B C D E 240 A B C D E

241 A B C D E 242 A B C D E 243 A B C D E 244 A B C D E 245 A B C D E 246 A B C D E 247 A B C D E 248 A B C D E

249 A B C D E 250 A B C D E 251 A B C D E 252 A B C D E 253 A B C D E 254 A B C D E 255 A B C D E 256 A B C D E

257 A B C D E 258 A B C D E 259 A B C D E 260 A B C D E 261 A B C D E 262 A B C D E 263 A B C D E 264 A B C D E

265 A B C D E 266 A B C D E 267 A B C D E 268 A B C D E 269 A B C D E 270 A B C D E 271 A B C D E 272 A B C D E

273 A B C D E 274 A B C D E 275 A B C D E 276 A B C D E 277 A B C D E 278 A B C D E 279 A B C D E 280 A B C D E

281 A B C D E 282 A B C D E 283 A B C D E 284 A B C D E 285 A B C D E 286 A B C D E 287 A B C D E 288 A B C D E

289 A B C D E 290 A B C D E 291 A B C D E 292 A B C D E 293 A B C D E 294 A B C D E 295 A B C D E 296 A B C D E

297 A B C D E 298 A B C D E 299 A B C D E 300 A B C D E 301 A B C D E 302 A B C D E 303 A B C D E 304 A B C D E

305 A B C D E 306 A B C D E 307 A B C D E 308 A B C D E 309 A B C D E 310 A B C D E 311 A B C D E 312 A B C D E

313 A B C D E 314 A B C D E 315 A B C D E 316 A B C D E 317 A B C D E 318 A B C D E 319 A B C D E 320 A B C D E